Intestinal Failure

Editor

ALAN L. BUCHMAN

GASTROENTEROLOGY
CLINICS OF NORTH AMERICA

www.gastro.theclinics.com

Consulting Editor
ALAN L. BUCHMAN

December 2019 • Volume 48 • Number 4

ELSEVIER

1600 John F. Kennedy Boulevard • Suite 1800 • Philadelphia, Pennsylvania, 19103-2899
http://www.theclinics.com

GASTROENTEROLOGY CLINICS OF NORTH AMERICA Volume 48, Number 4
December 2019 ISSN 0889-8553, ISBN-13: 978-0-323-69539-8

Editor: Kerry Holland
Developmental Editor: Laura Kavanaugh

Gastroenterology Clinics of North America (ISSN 0889-8553) is published quarterly by Elsevier Inc., 360 Park Avenue South, New York, NY 10010-1710. Months of issue are March, June, September, and December. Business and Editorial Offices: 1600 John F. Kennedy Blvd., Suite 1800, Philadelphia, PA 19103-2899. Customer Service Office: 6277 Sea Harbor Drive, Orlando, FL 32887-4800. Periodicals postage paid at New York, NY and additional mailing offices. Subscription prices are $361.00 per year (US individuals), $100.00 per year (US students), $692.00 per year (US institutions), $387.00 per year (Canadian individuals), $220.00 per year (Canadian students), $849.00 per year (Canadian institutions), $463.00 per year (international individuals), $220.00 per year (international students), and $849.00 per year (international institutions). Foreign air speed delivery is included in all *Clinics* subscription prices. All prices are subject to change without notice. **POSTMASTER**: Send address changes to *Gastroenterology Clinics of North America*, Elsevier Health Sciences Division, Subscription Customer Service, 3251 Riverport Lane, Maryland Heights, MO 63043. **Telephone: 1-800-654-2452 (U.S. and Canada); 314-447-8871 (outside U.S. and Canada). Fax: 314-447-8029. E-mail: journalscustomerservice-usa@elsevier.com (for print support); journalsonlinesupport-usa@elsevier.com (for online support)**.

Reprints. For copies of 100 or more, of articles in this publication, please contact the Commercial Reprints Department, Elsevier Inc., 360 Part Avenue South, New York, New York 10010-1710. Tel. 212-633-3874, Fax: 212-633-3820, E-mail: reprints@elsevier.com.

Gastroenterology Clinics of North America is also published in Italian by Il Pensiero Scientifico Editore, Rome, Italy; and in Portuguese by Interlivros Edicoes Ltda., Rua Commandante Coelho 1085, 21250 Cordovil, Rio de Janeiro, Brazil.

Gastroenterology Clinics of North America is covered in *MEDLINE/PubMed (Index Medicus), Excerpta Medica, Current Contents/Clinical Medicine, Science Citation Index, ISI/BIOMED,* and *BIOSIS.*

Contributors

CONSULTING EDITOR

ALAN L. BUCHMAN, MD, MSPH, FACP, FACN, FACG, AGAF
Medical Director, Health Care Services Corporation, Professor of Clinical Surgery, Medical Director, Intestinal Rehabilitation and Transplant Center, The University of Illinois at Chicago, UI Health, Department of Surgery, Chicago, Illinois, USA

EDITOR

ALAN L. BUCHMAN, MD, MSPH, FACP, FACN, FACG, AGAF
Medical Director, Health Care Services Corporation, Professor of Clinical Surgery, Medical Director, Intestinal Rehabilitation and Transplant Center, The University of Illinois at Chicago, UI Health, Department of Surgery, Chicago, Illinois, USA

AUTHORS

VALERIANNA K. AMOROSO, MD
Medical Director for Penn Home Infusion Therapy, University of Pennsylvania, Professor of Clinical Medicine, Perelman School of Medicine, Philadelphia, Pennsylvania, USA

JULIE M. ANDOLINA
Intern, The Oley Foundation, Albany Medical Center, Delmar, New York, USA

JOAN BISHOP
Executive Director, The Oley Foundation, Albany Medical Center, Delmar, New York, USA

VALERIA C. COHRAN, MD
Associated Professor of Pediatrics, Medical Director of Intestinal Rehabilitation and Transplant, Division of Gastroenterology, Hepatology, and Nutrition, Ann & Robert H. Lurie Children's Hospital of Chicago, Chicago, Illinois, USA

CONRAD R. COLE, MD
Professor of Pediatrics, University of Cincinnati College of Medicine, Medical Director, Intestinal Rehabilitation Program, Medical Director, Division of Gastroenterology, Hepatology, and Nutrition, Cincinnati Children's Hospital Medical Center, Cincinnati, Ohio, USA

RICCARDO COLLETTA, MD, PhD
Department of Paediatric Surgery, Center for Intestinal Reconstruction and Rehabilitation, Meyer Children's Hospital, Florence, Italy; School of Environment and Life Science, University of Salford, Salford, United Kingdom

CHARLENE COMPHER, PhD, RD, CNSC
Professor of Nutrition Science, University of Pennsylvania, School of Nursing, Philadelphia, Pennsylvania, USA

RACHEL COUGHLIN, MSN, RN
Manager of Quality and Patient Safety, Penn Home Infusion Therapy

PIETER DEMETTER, MD, PhD
Professor, Department of Pathology, Institut Bordet, Brussels, Belgium

DAVID J. HACKAM, MD, PhD
Garrett Professor and Chief of Pediatric Surgery, Professor of Surgery, Pediatrics and Cell Biology, Division of Pediatric Surgery, Johns Hopkins School of Medicine, Pediatric Surgeon-in-Chief and Co-Director, Johns Hopkins Children's Center, The Charlotte R. Bloomberg Children's Center, Johns Hopkins University, Baltimore, Maryland, USA

CIEL HARRIS, MD
Division of Gastroenterology, Department of Medicine, University of Florida Health, Jacksonville, Florida, USA

KISHORE IYER, MBBS, FRCS (Eng), FACS
Professor of Surgery and Pediatrics, Director, Intestinal Rehabilitation and Transplant Program, Icahn School of Medicine at Mount Sinai, Mount Sinai Hospital, New York, New York, USA

ARSHAD B. KAHN, MD, MS, MRCSed
General, Hepatobiliary and Transplant Surgeon, Director of Surgery at LifeCare Medical Center, Altru Health System, Roseau, Minnesota, USA

BRUCE P. KINOSIAN, MD
Associate Professor of Medicine, University of Pennsylvania, Perelman School of Medicine, Hospital of the University of Pennsylvania, Philadelphia, Pennsylvania, USA

MARK L. KOVLER, MD
Division of Pediatric Surgery, Johns Hopkins University, Johns Hopkins Children's Center, Baltimore, Maryland, USA

DANIEL LEVIN, MD
Assistant Professor of Surgery, Division of Pediatric Surgery, Department of Surgery, University of Virginia, Charlottesville, Virginia, USA

LISA CROSBY METZGER, BA
LifelineLetter Editor and Director of Community Engagement, The Oley Foundation, Albany Medical Center, Delmar, New York, USA

ETHAN A. MEZOFF, MD
Assistant Professor of Pediatrics, The Ohio State University College of Medicine, Center for Intestinal Rehabilitation and Nutrition Support, Division of Gastroenterology, Hepatology, and Nutrition, Nationwide Children's Hospital, Columbus, Ohio, USA

ANTONINO MORABITO, MD, FRCS
Professor and Director, Department of Paediatric Surgery, Center for Intestinal Reconstruction and Rehabilitation, Meyer Children's Hospital, Department of NeuroFarBa, University of Florence, Florence, Italy; School of Environment and Life Science, University of Salford, Salford, United Kingdom

OCTAVIA PICKETT-BLAKELY, MD, MHS
Director, GI Nutrition, Obesity and Celiac Disease Program, Division of Gastroenterology, University of Pennsylvania, Perelman School of Medicine, Assistant Professor of Clinical Medicine, Philadelphia, Pennsylvania, USA

LORIS PIRONI, MD
Professor, Chronic Intestinal Failure Unit, Department of Medical and Surgical Sciences, Saint Orsola Hospital, University of Bologna, Bologna, Italy

ANNA SIMONA SASDELLI, MD
Chronic Intestinal Failure Unit, Department of Medical and Surgical Sciences, Saint Orsola Hospital, University of Bologna, Bologna, Italy

PHYLLIS SCHIAVONE, MSN, CRNP
Advanced Practice Provider, Hospital of the University of Pennsylvania, Philadelphia, Pennsylvania, USA

JAMES S. SCOLAPIO, MD
Division of Gastroenterology, Associate Chair, Professor, Department of Medicine, University of Florida Health, Jacksonville, Florida, USA

NANCY EVANS STONER, MSN, RN
Nurse Clinical Specialist, Hospital of the University of Pennsylvania, Philadelphia, Pennsylvania, USA

KIARA A. TULLA, MD
Resident, Department of Surgery, University of Illinois at Chicago, Chicago, Illinois, USA

IVO G. TZVETANOV, MD, FACS
Associate Professor, Chief, Division of Transplantation, Department of Surgery, The University of Illinois at Chicago, Chicago, Illinois, USA

ANDREW UKLEJA, MD, AGAF
Lecturer in Medicine, Harvard Medical School, Division of Gastroenterology and Hepatology, Beth Israel Deaconess Medical Center/Beth Israel Lahey Health, Boston, Massachusetts, USA

ANDRÉ VAN GOSSUM, MD, PhD
Professor, Department of Gastroenterology, Hôpital Erasme/Institut Bordet, Université Libre de Bruxelles, Brussels, Belgium

ROBERT S. VENICK, MD
Professor of Pediatrics and Surgery, Division of Pediatric GI, Hepatology and Nutrition, David Geffen School of Medicine, UCLA, Director of Pediatric Liver and Intestinal Transplant Services, Mattel Children's Hospital UCLA, Los Angeles, California, USA

ZHIGANG XUE, MD
Peking Union Medical College Hospital, Peking Union Medical College, Beijing, China

Contents

Preface: Bringing Success to Intestinal Failure xiii

Alan L. Buchman

Initial Evaluation and Care of the Patient with New-Onset Intestinal Failure 465

Ciel Harris and James S. Scolapio

A total parenteral nutrition (TPN) formula needs to be correctly compounded with the help of a pharmacist and patients cycled to ensure they are tolerating the TPN volume. Selection of and close working relationship with a home infusion company needs to be arranged prior to hospital discharge and can be coordinated with the help of a hospital case manager. For Medicare patients, a certificate of medical necessity must be completed and signed prior to hospital discharge. Patients should undergo education regarding catheter care, infusion pump programming, and preparation of the TPN solution with additives, such as multivitamins and trace elements.

Preparing the Patient for Home Parenteral Nutrition and for a Successful Course of Therapy 471

Nancy Evans Stoner, Phyllis Schiavone, Bruce P. Kinosian, Octavia Pickett-Blakely, Valerianna K. Amoroso, Rachel Coughlin, Zhigang Xue, and Charlene Compher

Preparing the patient for home parenteral nutrition (HPN) is a collaborative effort among many different clinicians. Identifying patients who will transition home with parenteral nutrition (PN) as early as possible allows for a thoughtful and safe approach. Communication regarding the HPN goals is critical to the patient's success, whether the requirement for PN is temporary or permanent. Management of these complex patients is best served by a multidisciplinary team with expertise in the area of nutrition support. Adherence to available guidelines that define best practice is imperative in all aspects of care for the patient on HPN.

Etiology and Medical Management of Pediatric Intestinal Failure 483

Ethan A. Mezoff, Conrad R. Cole, and Valeria C. Cohran

Pediatric intestinal failure occurs when gut function is insufficient to meet the growing child's hydration and nutrition needs. After massive bowel resection, the remnant bowel adapts to lost absorptive and digestive capacity through incompletely defined mechanisms newly targeted for pharmacologic augmentation. Management seeks to achieve enteral autonomy and mitigate the development of comorbid disease. Care has improved, most notably related to reductions in blood stream infection and liver disease. The future likely holds expansion of pharmacologic adaptation augmentation, refinement of intestinal tissue engineering techniques, and the development of a learning health network for efficient multicenter study and care improvement.

Predictors of Intestinal Adaptation in Children   499

Robert S. Venick

In children, short-bowel syndrome (SBS) accounts for two-thirds of the cases of intestinal failure, and motility disorders and congenital mucosal diarrheal disorders account for the remaining one-third. Children with SBS are supported primarily by parenteral nutrition, which is the single-most important therapy contributing to their improved prognosis. More than 90% of children with SBS who are cared for at experienced intestinal rehabilitation programs survive, and roughly 60% to 70% undergo intestinal adaptation and achieve full enteral autonomy. This article focuses on the predictors of pediatric intestinal adaptation and discusses the pathophysiology and clinical management of children with SBS.

Management of the Patient with Chronic Intestinal Pseudo-Obstruction and Intestinal Failure   513

Loris Pironi and Anna Simona Sasdelli

Chronic intestinal pseudo-obstruction (CIPO) is a severe form of intestinal dysmotility disorder, characterized by the impairment of gastrointestinal propulsion of the gut content in the absence of fixed occluding lesions. CIPO is a rare disease that can develop in both children and adults. CIPO is classified as primary/idiopathic, when no underlying disorder is demonstrated, or secondary, when related to systemic diseases. Diagnosis relies on the finding of chronic/recurrent obstructive type symptoms with radiological features of dilated intestine with air/fluid levels without any lumen occluding lesion. Therapy is based on nutrition, pharmacologic and surgical intervention and requires a multidisciplinary approach.

Weaning from Parenteral Nutrition   525

Andrew Ukleja

The ultimate goal of treatment of short bowel syndrome/intestinal failure patients is to achieve enteral autonomy by eliminating parenteral nutrition (PN)/intravenous fluids (IV). After optimization of diet, oral hydration and anti-diarrheal medications, attempt should be made to eliminate PN/IV. Weaning from PN/IV should be individualized for each patient. Although teduglutide is the preferred agent for PN/IV volume reduction or successful weaning, optimal patient selection and long-term safety need further evaluation. Following PN/IV elimination, patients need long-term monitoring for nutritional deficiencies. This article will address clinical considerations before, during, and after PN/IV weaning to facilitate safe and successful PN/IV weaning process.

Hepatobiliary Complications of Chronic Intestinal Failure   551

André Van Gossum and Pieter Demetter

Intestinal failure-associated liver disease is a multifactorial process that may occur in patients with chronic intestinal failure on long-term home parenteral nutrition. A very short gut, the lack of enteral feeding, recurrent sepsis, and parenteral overfeeding are major risk factors. Histologic changes include steatosis, steatohepatitis, cholestasis, fibrosis, and cirrhosis. Chronic cholestasis is common, but does not always progress to fibrosis and/or cirrhosis. Preventing harmful factors may dramatically decrease the risk of intestinal failure-associated liver disease. Advanced liver disease is an indication for intestinal and/or multivisceral transplantation. Biliary stone formation is frequent and mainly due to a lack of enteral feeding.

Nontransplant Surgery for Intestinal Failure 565

Riccardo Colletta, Antonino Morabito, and Kishore Iyer

Insufficient absorptive mucosal surface is the fundamental problem in the short bowel state. Intestinal adaptation has been well studied, and it is well recognized that it may lead to dilatation of the bowel with increased thickness of the bowel wall, resulting from both mucosal hypertrophy and hyperplasia. Autologous reconstructive surgery exploits bowel dilatation in short bowel syndrome and maximizes the absorptive potential of the available mucosal surface. Indeed, autologous gastrointestinal reconstructive procedures may be better viewed as optimizing bowel diameter rather than focusing on length, thus allowing better prograde peristalsis and improved contact between luminal nutrients and mucosa, ultimately enhancing absorption.

Indications of Intestinal Transplantation 575

Arshad B. Kahn, Kiara A. Tulla, and Ivo G. Tzvetanov

The intestinal transplantation is reserved for patients with life-threatening complications of permanent intestinal failure or underlying gastrointestinal disease. The choice of the allograft for a particular patient depends on several factors and the presence of concurrent organ failure, and availability of the donor organs, and specialized care. Combined liver and intestinal transplant allows for patients who have parenteral nutrition–associated liver disease a possibility of improved quality of life and nutrition as well as survival. Intestinal transplantation has made giant strides over the past few decades to the present era where current graft survivals are comparable with other solid organ transplants.

Generating an Artificial Intestine for the Treatment of Short Bowel Syndrome 585

Mark L. Kovler and David J. Hackam

Intestinal failure is defined as the inability to maintain fluid, nutrition, energy, and micronutrient balance that leads to the inability to gain or maintain weight, resulting in malnutrition and dehydration. Causes of intestinal failure include short bowel syndrome (ie, the physical loss of intestinal surface area and severe intestinal dysmotility). For patients with intestinal failure who fail to achieve enteral autonomy through intestinal rehabilitation programs, the current treatment options are expensive and associated with severe complications. Therefore, the need persists for next-generation therapies, including cell-based therapy, to increase intestinal regeneration, and development of the tissue-engineered small intestine.

Bench to Bedside: Approaches for Engineered Intestine, Esophagus, and Colon 607

Daniel Levin

The generation of tissue engineered organs from autologous cells will allow replacement of diseased or absent organs without the need for immunosuppression. Common steps of tissue engineering include isolation of pluripotent or multipotent stem cells, preparation of synthetic or biologic scaffold, and implantation into a host to support the proliferation of engineered tissue. Some organs have been successfully transplanted in human patients; gastrointestinal tract tissues are nearing clinical introduction. The state of the science has progressed rapidly and providers and researchers alike must take appropriate steps to ensure strict adherence to ethical standards before introduction to human therapy.

The Oley Foundation and Consumer Support Groups 625

Julie M. Andolina, Lisa Crosby Metzger, and Joan Bishop

Patients with intestinal failure (IF) often require home parenteral and/or enteral nutrition (HPEN). There are many complications associated with both IF and the use of HPEN, including infection and intolerance. Psychosocial effects, such as depression, isolation, fatigue, anxiety, financial stress, are also associated with IF and HPEN and can be difficult to address. Support groups offer patients and caregivers the opportunity to talk to and learn from others who have had similar experiences. The Oley Foundation, a nonprofit organization for HPEN consumers, caregivers, and clinicians, fulfills the role of a traditional support group while offering many other resources and programs.

GASTROENTEROLOGY
CLINICS OF NORTH AMERICA

FORTHCOMING ISSUES

March 2020
Fatty Liver Disease
Arun J. Sanyal and Mohammad
Shadab Siddiqui, *Editors*

June 2020
Infections of Liver and Biliary Systems
K. Rajender Reddy, *Editor*

RECENT ISSUES

September 2019
The Microbiome: Interactions with Organ
Systems, Diet, and Genetics
Rochellys Dias Heijtz, *Editor*

June 2019
Laboratory Monitoring of Gastrointestinal
and Hepatobiliary Disease
Stanley J. Naides, *Editor*

SERIES OF RELATED INTEREST

Gastrointestinal Endoscopy Clinics of North America
(Available at: https://www.giendo.theclinics.com)
Clinics in Liver Disease
(Available at: https://www.liver.theclinics.com)

THE CLINICS ARE AVAILABLE ONLINE!
Access your subscription at:
www.theclinics.com

Preface

Bringing Success to Intestinal Failure

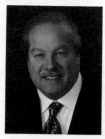

Alan L. Buchman, MD, MSPH
Editor

It is estimated there are approximately 25,000 patients, of which 20% are children, in the United States alone who require long-term, or home parenteral nutrition (PN) because of their inability to assimilate sufficient fluid or food through their digestive tract in order to maintain nutritional autonomy. In short, these patients, many with short bowel syndrome, excrete more fluid and energy in their stool than they consume. This heterogenous group of patients with varying disease states has 1 disease in common: intestinal failure. As such, they are perhaps the most challenging group of patients of any disease to manage successfully and gain quality of life. Therapy is expensive and highly technical and has numerous associated complications, although many of these are caused by the disease itself. Management of intestinal failure brings together ideas from around the world, hence, the international group of authors selected for this issue.

In this issue of *Gastroenterology Clinics of North America*, Drs Harris and Scolapio cover the initial evaluation and treatment of patients with intestinal failure once they have survived their catastrophic surgery or are first diagnosed with a severe malabsorptive disorder. Although not all of such patients will require longer-term PN in a rehabilitation facility or at home, the process of getting the patient ready medically, psychologically, and educationally is of obvious importance to ensure optimal outcome and minimize complications and hospital readmissions. The development of hepatic as well as biliary disease is a significant complication of intestinal failure, and indeed, intestinal failure–associated liver disease is the leading indication for small bowel transplants and is discussed by Drs Van Gossum and Demetter.

Children with intestinal failure are managed similarly to adults but have obvious and important nuances that are discussed by Drs Mezoff, Cole, Cohran, and Venick. With nutritional and pharmacologic therapy, the intestine, most notably in those with short bowel syndrome, adapts over time, and absorption becomes more efficient in both children and adults, as discussed by Dr Venick.

Gastroenterol Clin N Am 48 (2019) xiii–xiv
https://doi.org/10.1016/j.gtc.2019.08.013
0889-8553/19/© 2019 Published by Elsevier Inc.

Although the largest group of patients with intestinal failure manifests in short bowel syndrome, those with chronic intestinal pseudoobstruction syndrome represent the spectrum of motility disorders during which malabsorption may occur in relation to bacterial overgrowth and other factors. Management of these patients follows many of the principles that are important in other patients with intestinal failure, albeit it with some additional considerations, as discussed by Drs Pironi and Sasdelli.

Despite much of this issue being devoted to intestinal failure, comprising the management of such patients, the ultimate goal is to wean patients from intravenous feeding and fluid support. This can be accomplished by increasing oral and/or enteral intake, improving absorption efficiency, and adjusting diet in appropriate candidates and by various surgical procedures aimed at tapering dilated and dysfunctional intestine as well as intestinal transplantation. The medical and pharmacologic methods to wean patients from PN are discussed by Dr Ukleja. Nontransplant surgery, including the reanastomosis of the colon to residual small bowel to effect colonic carbohydrate salvage, as well as to surgically modify dilated loops of small bowel into functional absorptive segments, is discussed by Dr Iyer. Intestinal transplantation and its various flavors (isolated intestine, intestine liver, and variations of multivisceral transplantation) are discussed by Dr Tzvetanov. The penultimate goal is of course a natural intestinal construct that removes the need for PN support and intestinal transplantation, although the clinical reality of such is set in the future. The field is rapidly advancing though, as discussed by Drs Kovler, Hackman, and Levin.

The medical and surgical management of patient with intestinal failure cannot be successful without buy-in from the patients themselves, who need to learn and be trained in complex care techniques, many of which they will develop greater expertise at than hospital nurses who share in the care of their complications. Important in this educational and psychological commitment are patient support groups such as the Oley Foundation.

After reading through the 12 articles of this important issue, the reader should understand the complexity of the disease, intestinal failure, understand and apply basic medical and surgical management, and understand when such patients should be referred to select centers of expertise where both medical and surgical (nontransplant and transplant) modalities are available.

Alan L. Buchman, MD, MSPH
Intestinal Rehabilitation and Transplant Center
University of Illinois at Chicago
Chicago, IL 60612, USA

UI Health
Department of Surgery
840 South Wood Street
Suite 402 (MC958)
Chicago, IL 60612, USA

E-mail address:
a.buchman@hotmail.com

Initial Evaluation and Care of the Patient with New-Onset Intestinal Failure

Ciel Harris, MD, James S. Scolapio, MD*

KEYWORDS

- New-onset intestinal failure • Short bowel • Patient • Total parenteral nutrition

KEY POINTS

- A total parenteral nutrition (TPN) formula needs to be correctly compounded with the help of a pharmacist and patients cycled to ensure they are tolerating the TPN volume.
- The selection and close working relationship with a home infusion company needs to be arranged prior to hospital discharge and can be coordinated with the help of a hospital case manager.
- For Medicare patients, a certificate of medical necessity must be completed and signed by the treating physician prior to hospital discharge.
- Patients should undergo education regarding catheter care, infusion pump programming, and preparation of the TPN solution with additives, such as multivitamins and trace elements.

ANATOMY POST–SURGICAL RESECTION

The initial evaluation of a patient with short bowel syndrome is to determine the length and health of the remaining small intestine. Review of the surgical records provides this information. It also is necessary to determine if a patient has part of the colon remaining. This valuable information of a patient's anatomy provides prognostic information, including short-term and long-term fluid and nutritional requirements. The normal length of the small intestine is approximately 480 cm with a range of 300 cm to 800 cm. The large intestine is approximately 150 cm in length. The jejunum occupies the proximal two-fifths of the small intestine, and the ileum consists of the distal three-fifths, including the ileocecal valve, which slows small intestine fluid emptying into the colon. The gastrointestinal tract in healthy adults secretes approximately 4000 mL of fluid each day, which includes 500 mL of saliva, 2000 mL of gastric acid, and 1500 mL

Disclosures. None.
Division of Gastroenterology, Department of Medicine, University of Florida Health, 655 8th Street West, Jacksonville, FL 32209, USA
* Corresponding author.
E-mail address: James.Scolapio@jax.ufl.edu

Gastroenterol Clin N Am 48 (2019) 465–470
https://doi.org/10.1016/j.gtc.2019.08.001
0889-8553/19/© 2019 Elsevier Inc. All rights reserved.

gastro.theclinics.com

of pancreatic biliary secretions in response to approximately 3000 mL of oral food and drink consumed daily. Larger small intestine resections result in more significant losses of fluids and nutrients requiring more intravenous (IV) replacement. A patient with a proximal jejunostomy has higher losses of fluids, electrolytes, and nutrients compared with a patient with more remaining small intestine with an intact ileocecal value and colon remnant.

The terminal ileum also has the specialized function of absorbing bile salts and vitamin B_{12}. The dumping of bile salts into a colonic remnant may result in bile acid–induced diarrhea when more than 100 cm of the distal ileum is resected. If part of the colon is remaining, a high complex carbohydrate, low-fat diet may be beneficial to reduce diarrhea and increase nutrient absorption in the form of short-chain fatty acids.[1] In addition, in patients with a colonic remnant, a low oxalate oral diet reduces the risk of calcium oxalate absorption and subsequent renal stone formation. Experimental bile acid replacement also may increase the absorption of dietary fats and minimize weight loss in those patients with a colonic remnant.[2] Knowledge of the health of the remaining intestine also is important for prognostic information related to nutrient and fluid absorption in both the initial and long-term management of a patient with short bowel syndrome. For example, a diseased small intestine from Crohn disease or radiation enteritis adversely affects absorption of fluids and nutrients.

The distal 50 cm to 60 cm of ileum is also the primary site for absorption of vitamin B_{12}, bound to intrinsic factor. Resection of the terminal ileum is associated with malabsorption of vitamin B_{12} and can lead to clinical deficiency unless supplemented. The distal ileum also is the selective location for absorption bile acids. In adults, resection of greater than 100 cm of terminal ileum leads to a disturbance of the enterohepatic circulation, ultimately resulting in bile acid deficiency because bile acid losses exceed the compensatory increase in hepatic bile acid production.[2] The diminished bile acid pool decreases the absorption of dietary fat and fat-soluble vitamins. In addition, the increased passage of bile acids into the colon may result in a colonic secretomotor diarrhea, known as choleretic enteropathy. Malabsorption of bile acids also leads to increased absorption of oxalate, leading to hyperoxaluria, which increases the risk of oxalate renal stones and risk of chronic kidney disease. Patients with short bowel syndrome without an ileum also lose the beneficial effects of the ileal brake, resulting in a rapid transit and decreased absorption of nutrients and fluids. The ileum normally reabsorbs a large portion of the fluid secreted by the jejunum during the digestive process, which is particularly important with the large intake of oral fluids or hypertonic feedings. This subset of short bowel patients often cannot tolerate large bolus feedings or diets of high osmolality, including high concentrations of simple carbohydrates.[1,3]

The ileocecal valve protects against the reflux of colonic material from the colon into the small intestine, preventing potential bacterial overgrowth.[4,5] Resection of the ileocecal valve also deceases the ability to wean patients off parenteral nutrition and IV fluids. This is likely due to a decrease in the small intestinal transit time, leading to an impairment of nutrient and fluid absorption.

Compared with the rest of the intestine, the colon has the slowest transit but greatest efficiency in the absorption of sodium and water. Approximately 10% of the fluid that enters the colon is absorbed. In patients with extensive bowel resections, more fluid exits the small intestine, which can then be absorbed by the colon. Additionally, the colon absorbs up to 15% of the body's daily requirements mainly in the form of short-chain fatty acids. This explains the positive effect of a high complex carbohydrate diet in those patients with part of their colon remaining.

INTRAVENOUS FLUID AND ELECTROLYTE MANAGEMENT POSTOPERATIVELY

There is no consensus in the management of acute intestinal failure with a specific fluid or electrolyte solution. Appropriate IV fluid and electrolyte replacement is the fundamental strategy after intestinal resection.[2] IV fluid replacement should be initiated prior to total parenteral nutrition (TPN) infusion. Fluids should be infused to cover all measured losses, including urine and stool output. Ongoing assessment and monitoring of patients output to determine their fluid and electrolyte status are important before, during, and after IV fluid resuscitation. Frequently encountered abnormalities in the immediate postoperative period include hypochloremia, hypokalemia metabolic alkalosis with paradoxic aciduria, and poor tissue perfusion, leading to lactic acidosis. Nonanion gap acidosis due to bicarbonate loss in stoma output, a blood urea nitrogen:creatinine ratio greater than 20:1, and other significant laboratory abnormalities, including low magnesium levels, can occur. During IV fluid and electrolyte replacement, it is important to monitor for signs of fluid overload, with specific attention given to those patients with heart, liver, and kidney disease.

Isotonic saline is one of the most commonly used IV solutions.[6,7] The normal daily requirement of sodium is 70 mmol to 100 mmol and 1 L of 0.9% saline contains approximately 154 mmol. Patients with intestinal failure with high-output gastrointestinal losses benefit the most from additional electrolyte replacement. These intestinal losses can be high in potassium, calcium, and magnesium. IV lactate ringers also are a reasonable alternative to normal saline. A study of critically ill adults showed no difference in hospital-free days between normal saline and lactate ringers; however, lactate ringers reported a lower incidence of major adverse kidney events at 30 days.[6] This study was performed in emergency room patients with normal baseline electrolytes; therefore, it is difficult to extrapolate results to those patients with intestinal failure.

Although it is important to effectively replace electrolytes and fluids IV, oral hydration therapy should be considered as well. Oral glucose and sodium solutions are absorbed by passive diffusion, which results in water absorption from the small intestine. This physiologic mechanism is referred to as solvent drag. This basic physiologic principle is important because the jejunum is permeable to both sodium and chloride. Oral solutions with a high sodium and chloride content result in increased water absorption. Oral rehydration solutions are less helpful in those patients who have had large resections of jejunum, because water absorption in the ileum is less efficient. Oral rehydration solutions also are beneficial patients with part of their part of their colons remaining. Many commercial oral rehydration formulas are available.

Enteral nutrition should be considered in the immediate postoperative period because it has trophic effects on the small intestine, may increase intestinal adaptation or growth, and may prevent bacterial translocation.[8] Patients should be counseled to avoid hypertonic fluids, such as soda and fruit juices, because they can cause osmotic diarrhea, which worsens fluid losses. In addition, hypotonic fluids, such as excess water, tea, coffee, and alcohol, do not contain the optimum concentrations of sodium or glucose necessary to facilitate absorption in patients with end jejunostomy and may lead to dehydration if consumed in large amounts. Patients with a residual colon can usually maintain adequate hydration without excessive fluid loss using these hypotonic fluids.

HYPERGASTRIC ACID SECRETION

Gastric acid hypersecretion occurs after larger resections of the small intestine. Increased gastric acid secretion can result in peptic ulcer disease as well as deactivation of pancreatic enzymes. Decreased pancreatic enzyme function decreases the optimal pH necessary for fat absorption. Hypersecretion of gastric acid secretions and subsequent fluid losses result in increased ostomy output. Gastric acid hypersecretion usually occurs for 1 year post–intestinal resection. Management includes fluid replacement and IV or oral acid blockade. An oral proton pump inhibitor, or high-dose histamine receptor type 2 antagonist, usually is beneficial in reducing fluid losses. Proton pump inhibitors also have been shown to directly increase water absorption and are most beneficial in those patients with ostomy output greater than 2.5 L a day.[9] Proton pump inhibitors and histamine-2 antagonist can be administered concomitantly for improved gastric acid secretion control. Histamine-2 antagonists can be added to the TPN solutions, unlike proton pump inhibitors, which ae not compatible with the solution.

DIARRHEA MEASUREMENT AND MANAGEMENT USING ANTIDIARRHEALS

Oral antidiarrheal medications are helpful in reducing intestinal fluid and electrolyte losses after intestinal resection. Medications commonly used include loperamide (Imodium), atropine/diphenoxylate (Lomotil), tincture of opium, clonidine, and octreotide.[2,3] Loperamide usually is the first choice because it is has no central nervous system side effects. Larger oral doses can be given safely and effectively, with the understanding that not all the medication is absorbed in patients with short bowel syndrome. Patients can be advised to open the capsules and mix the contents with meals to help increase absorption. Loperamide usually is administered as 4 mg to 6 mg orally 4 times daily. With larger resections, higher oral doses, such as 16 mg, may be helpful. The does can be titrated to control stool output to under 2 L a day. Reducing the amount of diarrhea usually helps with a patient's overall quality of life. In those patients without a colon or those who have a minimum length of remaining jejunum or duodenum, medications, such as codeine sulfate and tincture of opium, may be helpful. Codeine and tincture of opium are absorbed across the blood-brain barrier and side effects include drowsiness, which limit its use. These medications have a longer duration of action and work at a different intestinal receptor than loperamide. Use of codeine or tincture of opium with loperamide seems to have a synergistic effect. Although gastrointestinal fluid losses decrease with antidiarrheal medications, positive water balance is rarely achieved. Octreotide is a somatostatin analogue that inhibits the release of growth hormone and various gastrointestinal and pancreatic hormones. It reduces the secretion of gastric fluids and increases the absorption of water and electrolytes. Octreotide typically is reserved for patients with a proximal jejunostomy and stool losses greater than 2 L a day. Octreotide decreases splanchnic protein synthesis, thereby potentially decreasing the normal intestinal adaptation process. There also is an increased incidence of gallbladder sludge and gallstone formation; therefore, long-term use is not recommended. Transdermal clonidine patch is another medication that can be used in patients with short bowel syndrome. Clonidine works as an antidiarrheal by its effects on chloride and water absorption.[10] Potential side effect include hypotension, rebound hypertension, and dry mouth. Clonidine was reported to be effective in refractory diarrhea in patients who have failed other antidiarrheal treatments. Glucagon-like peptide-1 and peptide-2 analogues are reported to significantly reduce fecal wet weight and intestinal losses compared with placebo and are discussed in Riccardo Colletta's article, "Non-transplant Surgery for Intestinal Failure," in this issue.[11]

TOTAL PARENTERAL NUTRITION MANAGEMENT AND CYCLING PRIOR TO DISCHARGE

TPN typically is started 3 days to 5 days postoperatively, provided the patient is not fluid overloaded and is hemodynamically stable. A single lumen subclavian vein catheter or a peripherally inserted central catheter should be placed for venous access. Before infusion, proper insertion of the catheter tip in the superior vena cava should be confirmed by chest radiograph. TPN typically is given as a 2-L solution containing carbohydrate, protein, and lipid. A pharmacist knowledgeable in TPN compounding should be consulted for the appropriate TPN mixture.[12] Before infusing, caution needs to be given to those patients who are severely dehydrated and fluid overloaded. Refeeding syndrome is a risk in patients who are severely malnourished. In patients at risk of refeeding syndrome, TPN should be increased slowly to the target infusion rate. The infusion rate of a 2-L TPN solution is based on a 24-hour infusion period. Infusion should be started at half the goal rate, 40 mL/h, and then advanced to the target rate, 80 mL/h, over 48 hours, as tolerated. Serum electrolytes should be checked at least twice a week and blood glucose levels should be checked daily until stable. If blood glucose levels are greater than 200 mg/dL, regular insulin can be added to the TPN solution to maintain glucose levels under 200 mg/dL. Prior to hospital discharge, the TPN infusion should be cycled from a 24-hour infusion period to approximately a 10-hour to 12-hour infusion period, typically over 3 days and during a patient's normal sleeping hours. It is important to document that the patient is tolerating the volume of TPN fluid infusion during the cycling process and prior to hospital discharge. Administering TPN infusion during normal sleep hours allows a patient autonomy with normal daytime activities. In addition, cycling TPN promotes appetite compared with a continuous infusion. Cycled TPN also minimizes high levels of insulin secretion, which may minimize hepatic steatosis and subsequent liver disease.

HOME PARENTERAL NUTRITION

The cornerstone of efficient and effective home parenteral nutrition delivery prior to hospital discharge relies on a multidisciplinary team consisting of a physician, nurse, dietician, pharmacist, and case manager.[13] The TPN formula needs to be compounded correctly with the help of a pharmacist and patients cycled to ensure they are tolerating the TPN volume. The selection and close working relationship with a home infusion company needs to be arranged prior to hospital discharge and can be coordinated with the help of the hospital case manager. For Medicare patients, a certificate of medical necessity must be completed and signed by the treating physician prior to hospital discharge. Patients should undergo education regarding catheter care, infusion pump programming, and preparation of the TPN solution with additives, such as multivitamins and trace elements. Patients also need to be taught to recognition acute complications, such as hypoglycemia and fever, which is often associated with the IV catheter and blood stream infection. Education by the nursing staff on sterile catheter technique and catheter hook-up and disconnect is important prior to hospital discharge. Catheter sepsis in the most common complication of TPN and can be life-threatening if not treated early with IV antibiotics. Catheter sepsis rate is approximately 0.13 episodes per year.[13] Laboratory testing initially should 'be done once a week after hospital discharge and then decreased to once a month after the patient has adjusted to the TPN infusion. Trace elements (manganese, copper, chromium, selenium, and zinc), fat-soluble vitamins (vitamins A, D, E, and K), and liver function tests should be checked approximately every 6 months.

REFERENCES

1. Pironi L, Arends J, Baxter J, et al. ESPEN endorsed recommendations. Definition and classification of intestinal failure in adults. Clin Nutr 2015;34(2):171–80.
2. O'Keefe SJ, Buchman AL, Fishbein TM, et al. Short bowel syndrome and intestinal failure: consensus definitions and overview. Clin Gastroenterol Hepatol 2006;4:6.

3. Thompson JS, Rochling FA, Weseman RA, et al. Current management of short bowel syndrome. Curr Probl Surg 2012;49:52.
4. Hofmann AF, Poley JR. Role of bile acid malabsorption in pathogenesis of diarrhea and steatorrhea in patients with ileal resection. I. Response to cholestyramine or replacement of dietary long chain triglyceride by medium chain triglyceride. Gastroenterology 1972;62:918.
5. Dibaise JK, Young RJ, Vanderhoof JA. Enteric microbial flora, bacterial overgrowth, and short-bowel syndrome. Clin Gastroenterol Hepatol 2006;4:11.
6. Semler MW, Self WH, Wanderer JP, et al. Balanced crystalloids versus saline in critically ill adults. N Engl J Med 2018;378(9):829–39.
7. Marjanovic G, Villain C, Timme S, et al. Colloid vs. crystalloid infusions in gastrointestinal surgery and their different impact on the healing of intestinal anastomoses. Int J Colorectal Dis 2010;25:491–8.
8. Lewis SJ, Egger M, Sylvester PA, et al. Early enteral feeding versus "nil by mouth" after gastrointestinal surgery: systematic review and meta-analysis of controlled trials. BMJ 2001;323(7316):773–6.
9. Jeppesen PB, Staun M, Tjellesen L, et al. Effect of intravenous ranitidine and omeprazole on intestinal absorption of water, sodium, and macronutrients in patients with intestinal resection. Gut 1998;43(6):763–9.
10. Fragkos KC, Zárate-Lopez N, Frangos CC. What about clonidine for diarrhoea? A systematic review and meta-analysis of its effect in humans. Therap Adv Gastroenterol 2016;9(3):282–301.
11. Madsen KB, Askov-Hansen C, Naimi RM, et al. Acute effects of continuous infusions of glucagon-like peptide (GLP)-1, GLP-2 and the combination (GLP-1+GLP-2) on intestinal absorption in short bowel syndrome (SBS) patients. A placebo-controlled study. Regul Pept 2013;184:30.
12. Boullata JI, Gilbert K, Sacks G, et al. A.S.P.E.N. clinical guidelines: parenteral nutrition ordering, order review, compounding, labeling, and dispensing. JPEN J Parenter Enteral Nutr 2014;38:334.
13. Staun M, Pironi L, Bozzetti F, et al. ESPEN guidelines on parenteral nutrition: Home Parenteral Nutrition (HPN) in adult patients. Clin Nutr 2009;28:467–79.

Preparing the Patient for Home Parenteral Nutrition and for a Successful Course of Therapy

Nancy Evans Stoner, MSN, RN[a], Phyllis Schiavone, MSN, CRNP[a],
Bruce P. Kinosian, MD[a], Octavia Pickett-Blakely, MD, MHS[b],
Valerianna K. Amoroso, MD[c], Rachel Coughlin, MSN, RN[d],
Zhigang Xue, MD[e], Charlene Compher, PhD, RD, CNSC[f],*

KEYWORDS

- Home parenteral nutrition • Short-bowel syndrome • Dysmotility • Malnutrition
- Bowel obstruction • Quality of life

KEY POINTS

- Early identification of patients who require home parenteral nutrition eases the transition home.
- Multidisciplinary home parenteral nutrition teams can provide a feasible, effective course of therapy.
- Selecting the best venous access device for the patient's needs is vitally important.
- Obtaining insurance coverage for the course of therapy can relieve the patient's or caregiver's anxiety about health care costs.
- Training for safe management of home parenteral nutrition in the patient's home enables assessment of the site and patient skill level.

INTRODUCTION

Home Parenteral Nutrition in the United States

Malnutrition is associated with many of the acute and chronic diseases treated in hospitals in the United States. During the course of a hospital admission, parenteral

Disclosure Statement: None.
[a] Hospital of the University of Pennsylvania, 3400 Spruce Street, Philadelphia, PA 19104, USA;
[b] GI Nutrition, Obesity and Celiac Disease Program, Division of Gastroenterology, University of Pennsylvania Perelman School of Medicine, 3400 Spruce Street, Philadelphia, PA 19104, USA;
[c] University of Pennsylvania, Perelman School of Medicine, 3400 Spruce Street, Philadelphia, PA 19104, USA; [d] Penn Home Infusion Therapy; [e] Peking Union Medical College Hospital, Peking Union Medical College, Beijing, China; [f] University of Pennsylvania, School of Nursing, 418 Curie Boulevard, Philadelphia, PA 19104-4217, USA
* Corresponding author.
E-mail address: compherc@upenn.edu

Gastroenterol Clin N Am 48 (2019) 471–481
https://doi.org/10.1016/j.gtc.2019.08.002
0889-8553/19/© 2019 Elsevier Inc. All rights reserved.

nutrition (PN) may be initiated for patients who either do not tolerate enteral nutrition or whose bowel function is so limited that they cannot obtain adequate nutrients and fluid by the oral route. A decision may be made to continue the PN in the patient's home after hospital discharge, thus initiating home PN (HPN) care.

Actual prevalence data for HPN in the United States are not available. However, based on analysis of government insurance data (Centers for Medicare and Medicaid Services) from 2013 and comparison with shared data from 3 of the largest home infusion pharmacy providers, approximately 25,000 adult patients were projected to receive HPN in 2013.[1] Approximately 27% of these patients received HPN financed by government insurance. This current estimate is considerably below the estimate made in 1992 using a similar approach.[2]

The Penn Clinical Nutrition Support HPN team provides care management for approximately 120 patients each month, more than 300 unique patients in fiscal year 2018. Approximately 15 new patients are initiated on HPN therapy each month. Our current population of HPN patients includes a range of HPN therapy experience, with a median HPN duration of 13 months (range 1 month to 28 years).

Common Indications for Home Parenteral Nutrition

Patients with severe intestinal failure may require either a short or lifetime course of HPN. The American Society for Parenteral and Enteral Nutrition (ASPEN) Sustain Registry of HPN patients included data from 1064 adult and 187 pediatric HPN patients.[3] Of these 1251 patients, the most common diagnoses were short-bowel syndrome (SBS), gastrointestinal obstruction or fistula, motility disorder, malabsorption, and intractable vomiting (**Table 1**).[3] Patients with a short course of therapy may have a surgical complication that is expected to be corrected after a period of HPN or potentially as a component of end-of-life care. Patients with the expectation of lifelong care are more likely to have SBS or a dysmotility disorder.

Our HPN service is represented in **Fig. 1**. The most common diagnoses are SBS, cancer, and dysmotility. Shorter-term episodes of care are provided for patients with malnutrition, Crohn disease, surgical complications, or bowel obstruction.

THE BENEFITS OF A MULTIDISCIPLINARY NUTRITION SUPPORT TEAM IN HOME PARENTERAL NUTRITION MANAGEMENT

The Penn Hospital–based nutrition support team is composed of 2 advanced practice nurse providers, an internist physician who has a specialty in nutrition support, a PharmD, and a clinical dietitian specialist. The physician and one of the advanced practice nurses is on call at all times as a resource for patient questions, problems, and response to extreme laboratory results.

Other regular collaborators are a gastroenterologist, an infectious disease physician, a nurse who is a manager of patient quality and safety for the infusion company, and 2 nurse liaisons who work in the hospital providing the first level of training. The home infusion company also provides infusion nurses for patient training at home and for catheter care and blood draw visits.

COMMUNICATION IS AN ESSENTIAL COMPONENT TO SUCCESSFUL DISCHARGE WITH HOME PARENTERAL NUTRITION

The advanced practice nurses begin this important function by identifying the important individuals to support the course of HPN and how best to contact them (**Box 1**). Shared goals about the course of therapy are also gathered in early in-hospital visits. Communication continues to be an essential component of the support of a patient

Table 1
Indications for home parenteral nutrition among adult patients (n = 1064) enrolled in the Sustain Registry between August 2011 and February 2014

Diagnosis or Clinical Condition	n	%
Short-bowel syndrome	250	24
Gastrointestinal obstruction	248	23
Gastrointestinal fistula	198	19
Gastrointestinal motility disorder	110	10
Non–short-bowel syndrome diarrhea/malabsorption	101	10
Intractable vomiting	60	9
Enteral feeding intolerance	55	9
Active inflammatory bowel disease	31	3
Malnutrition	31	3
Chemotherapy-associated gastrointestinal dysfunction	29	3
Pancreatitis	24	2
Intractable diarrhea	19	2
Gastrointestinal perforation or leak	17	2
Radiation enteritis	13	1
Anastomotic ulcer or stricture	10	1
Chyle leak	10	1
Mesenteric ischemia	10	1
Abscess	8	<1
Gastrointestinal cancer	6	<1
Gastric ulcer	3	<0.5
Graft versus host disease	3	<0.5
Congenital bowel defect	2	<0.5
Neurologic swallowing disorder	2	<0.5
Other	15	1

Patients may have multiple indications for home parenteral nutrition.
From Winkler MF, DiMaria-Ghalili RA, Guenter P, et al. Characteristics of a Cohort of Home Parenteral Nutrition Patients at the Time of Enrollment in the Sustain Registry. *JPEN J Parenter Enteral Nutr.* 2016;40(8):1140-1149; with permission.

once home with therapy, although the communication includes other health providers in an effort to include the HPN care in the patient's overall medical care.

SECURING INSURANCE COVERAGE FOR HOME PARENTERAL NUTRITION

To obtain insurance coverage for HPN often requires documentation of medical necessity for the therapy. Careful and detailed documentation of the medical or surgical diagnosis that limits gastrointestinal (GI) function to the extent that HPN is needed is necessary. If the patient is not required to be without any intake by mouth (NPO), then documentation of failed enteral tube feedings may be needed or some evidence of malabsorption. A projected HPN course of at least 3 months in duration is usual other than for a planned corrective surgical procedure for which a shorter duration may be appropriate. For patients with longer-term diagnoses of SBS and dysmotility, the prognosis of lifelong HPN should be stated at the outset of HPN therapy even when efforts to reduce days of infusion are planned.

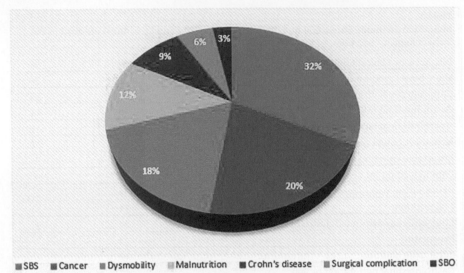

■ SBS   ■ Cancer   ■ Dysmobility   ▨ Malnutrition   ■ Crohn's disease   ■ Surgical complication   ■ SBO

Fig. 1. Penn HPN patients by proportion of diagnostic groups. SBO, small bowel obstruction.

SELECTION OF CENTRAL VASCULAR ACCESS DEVICE

Several types of central vascular access device (CVAD) are available for use in HPN patients. The peripherally inserted central catheter (PICC) may have 1 to 3 lumens. Tunneled CVADs are held in place by a cuff within the tunnel to anchor the CVAD and prevent microbial migration into the venous system, and typically have 1 or 2 lumens. Implanted CVADs are fully covered by the patient's skin but require the insertion of a needle for infusion. To minimize the risk of infection, a CVAD with the fewest number of lumens should be placed.[4] When multiple therapies are required (such as chemotherapy or antibiotics) and a multilumen catheter is placed, it is important to reserve 1 lumen for the PN infusion to avoid interruption of the HPN and reduce infection risk.[5]

The procedure required to place the catheter varies. The PICC may be placed at the bedside by a trained nurse or by a radiologist. Tunneled and implanted CVADs may be placed in the radiology suite or in the operating room.

Table 2 illustrates key considerations about the choice of type of CVAD.[6] A key consideration in the type of catheter selected for HPN patients is the length of therapy that is anticipated. The ASPEN guideline for adult HPN patients suggests tunneled CVADs for patients who require daily long-term infusions, based on weak evidence.[6] However, they recognize that for HPN of uncertain or short duration, a PICC may be used.

Patient and caregiver preferences also should be considered in the decision about type of CVAD. Patients who want the freedom to swim may prefer an implanted CVAD, as there is no risk of contamination of the catheter by bacteria in the swimming pool. Patients who participate in active sports may find the PICC inconvenient because of the risk of catheter dislodgement. The location of the exit site is an important consideration in order for patients to be independent with infusion procedures. Before catheter placement, we take time to discuss this with the patient and may mark a proposed exit site on the patient that the patient can easily access. Patient and caregiver ability are especially important with implanted CVADs, as the needle may need to be

---

Box 1
Important communications bullet list

Communications with the patient:

- Patient telephone, e-mail, and preferred means of contact
- Family caregivers
- Medical providers including the primary physician and any needed consultants
- Goals of home parenteral nutrition (HPN) care based on anatomy, disease process
- Likely duration of therapy
- Patient's goal weight
- Patient's comfort with the mechanical, technological, and infection control aspects of HPN infusion independently or with a designated caregiver
- The need for stable electrolyte, hydration and glycemic management as parenteral nutrition is cycled over 12 hours
- HPN supplier and nursing service with contact information
- Contact information for the hospital-based HPN team

Communications with others on the patient's behalf

- An initial letter documenting the patient's discharge with HPN and contact information from team providers is sent immediately after discharge to collaborating physicians and posted in the electronic medical record (EMR).
- Letters reflecting the findings from outpatient clinic visits are sent to collaborating physician groups and posted in the EMR.
- The nurse's evaluation of the patient's progress with the initiation of HPN, ongoing tracking of issues or concerns, and the results of weekly monitoring of laboratory values (in collaboration with the ordering physician and other team members) with the patient by telephone call are documented in the EMR.
- Any needed modifications to the HPN orders are communicated to the HPN supplier, to the patient, and documented in the EMR.
- Travel letters on hospital letterhead are supplied to enable patients who travel to pass airport security stations carrying any needed supplies. Patients are also provided with additional information about handling of the catheter during unusual situations such as swimming in the ocean. When patients need access to a local HPN expert while traveling, team members locate a suitable provider with contact information and communication to the provider of the HPN team contact if patient information is required.

---

replaced by the patient or caregiver more frequently than a home infusion nurse can come to assist.

The type of CVAD used by the Penn HPN service varies by expected duration of therapy and by overall management after a central line–associated bloodstream infection (CLABSI). When patients are destined for lifelong HPN therapy, a tunneled catheter or implanted port is preferred. The PICC is often placed to facilitate preparation for initial discharge with HPN. The PICC may also be placed after removal of a CVAD due to CLABSI, with an intention of replacement of the PICC with a tunneled or implanted CVAD at some later time. Patients dependent on HPN for many years are at a greater risk for limited vascular access. In these patients, the traditional approach to CVAD placement is often compromised and translumbar or femoral catheters are used. Exit sites for these catheters should be kept away from the groin area or from ostomy appliances to reduce the potential for infection. Although our goal is generally to use a

Table 2
Types of central vascular access devices for HPN

Type	Dwell Time	Therapeutic Applications	PN Considerations
PICCs	Maximum dwell time is unknown.	Suitable for acute care and short-term and medium-term PN for adults and pediatric patients.	Associated with an increased risk for deep vein thrombosis, limiting use for indefinite PN therapy and situations in which vessel preservation is a priority. Antecubital location of exit site hinders self-care and activity. Clothing may not always cover insertion site, potentially having a negative impact on body image; may be easily removed when infected or PN is no longer needed.
Tunneled CVADs (Hickman, Broviac, Hohn types)	3 months–years	Suitable for long-term PN; the presence of a cuff within the tunnel inhibits microbial migration and decreases risk of dislodgement.	No restrictions on upper extremity activity; position on chest facilitates self-care; VAD can be easily hidden under clothing.
Implanted ports	6 months–years	Primarily intended for low-frequency, intermittent access. Associated with lowest risk for CLABSI due to reduced manipulation. The presence of an indwelling needle to continuous or frequent access offsets the reduced infection benefit.	Suitable for PN in selected circumstances; motivated patients can learn access procedures; body image remains intact; requires no local site care when device is not accessed. PN may increase risk for CLABSI and occlusion in children with cancer.

Abbreviations: CLABSI, central line–associated bloodstream infection; CVAD, central vascular access device; HPN, home parenteral nutrition; PICC, peripherally inserted central catheter; PN, parenteral nutrition; VAD, vascular access device.

From Kovacevich DS, Corrigan M, Ross VM, McKeever L, Hall AM, Braunschweig C. American Society for Parenteral and Enteral Nutrition Guidelines for the Selection and Care of Central Venous Access Devices for Adult Home Parenteral Nutrition Administration. *JPEN J Parenter Enteral Nutr.* 2019;43(1):15-31; with permission.

PICC for shorter courses of HPN, some patients planned for short courses may actually require longer care. Some patients also manage a PICC without experiencing a CLABSI for prolonged periods and are not inclined to change to a different type. The choice of CVAD once again is negotiated among the HPN team, the physician placing the new CVAD, and the patient.

PREPARING A HOME NUTRIENT PRESCRIPTION

Although many patients receive PN over 24 hours during their hospital stay, patients preparing for discharge on HPN are more typically supported with a shorter infusion time, a cycled infusion. Once the patient is receiving the goal nutrient prescription and serum electrolytes and blood glucose levels are stable, the PN infusion time can be reduced from 24 to 16 and finally to 12 hours. This progression will typically take an average of 1 to 3 days, and is an expectation for most home infusion providers to accept the patient. Although the hospital standard for cycling PN may be a nocturnal infusion, occasional patients at home may prefer a daytime cycle as a strategy to facilitate nighttime sleep or glycemic control. Glycemic control also may be eased in some patients with infusion over a longer 16-hour than shorter cycled infusion time.

The initial HPN orders may differ from that provided during the hospital admission in terms of volume delivered. Patients with excessive GI fluid losses may have additional intravenous (IV) fluid replacement in addition to the PN regimen while hospitalized. However, for the patient's therapy at home, it is preferable to combine all needed fluid into a single infusion to run typically overnight. Because the current maximum volume of infusion bags is 4 L, patients with extreme GI losses may also require additional saline infusion at times outside the HPN infusion time.

The amino acid and energy content of the HPN regimen may require adjustment. Hospitalized patients initiating HPN may be very catabolic and require high doses of amino acids. As they recover and approach discharge, these needs often can be adjusted and protein delivery reduced. The proportion of dextrose in an HPN solution may be varied depending on glycemic control and patient tolerance to IV fat emulsion (IVFE). Regardless, maximal intake of 7 g/kg per day dextrose should not be exceeded. The standard soy-based solution IVFE can be provided if the patient is not allergic to eggs or soy. If the patient is not allergic to fish, egg, soy, or peanuts, a 4-oil IVFE (Smoflipid; Fresenius-Kabi, Lake Zurich, IL) has been approved by the Food and Drug Administration and is now available in the United States for adult patients. This IVFE product has been used for many years in other global markets and contains soybean oil, medium chain triglycerides, olive oil, and fish oil. Smoflipid might be considered for patients with transaminitis or hyperbilirubinemia. Regardless, an upper limit of 1 g fat emulsion/kg per day should be used. The lipid doses may be given over only a few days weekly.

Although the goal for most hospitalized PN patients in terms of electrolyte management is to replace variable and potentially excessive losses, the goal for HPN patients is to provide electrolyte stability (in spite of GI losses) for at least 1 week of HPN orders. Some patients do well with a standard electrolyte regimen, whereas others with excess losses need additional magnesium, zinc, potassium, phosphorus, or calcium.

Standard intake of trace elements are added to the HPN solution during preparation by the HPN supplier, but provision of vitamins requires patient or caregiver skill. Parenteral multivitamins are added by the patient to the solution just before infusion to avoid losses from light exposure. Any additional vitamin preparations are individual patient additions to the solution and increase the complexity of their regimen, add to potential for error, and heighten the risk of infusion contamination. If the patient is at risk for vitamin B_{12} deficiency due to loss of the terminal ileum with bowel resection, monthly B_{12} injections can be ordered and administered in the home.

The full HPN program may also include IV antibiotics to complete treatment that was started during the hospital admission. The simplest antibiotic regimen that will be effective should be considered, as each dose requires an additional contact with the catheter. The frequency of antibiotic therapy should be no more than twice daily if possible to avoid interruption of the PN infusion.[4] Patients receive training by the home infusion nurse with each new IV antibiotic order.

PATIENT EDUCATION AND TRAINING

HPN teaching begins before hospital discharge (**Box 2**). Nurse liaisons meet with the patient and/or caregiver to provide hands-on instruction on the infusion-related equipment and technique. The equipment instruction includes management of the HPN pump (inserting the battery, turning the pump on and off, starting the infusion, and troubleshooting common pump alarms). Infusion technique instruction includes spiking an empty total PN (TPN) bag, connecting and disconnecting the TPN tubing cassette to the pump, cleaning the injection cap of the central line access site, bathing without risk to the catheter, recognizing air in the line, and contacting the home infusion company with any questions. This in-hospital education is designed to provide a foundation for the home infusion nurse to build on after discharge.

At each of 3 home visits, the infusion nurse will reiterate the pump education as well as hand washing; gathering needed supplies before beginning TPN infusion; review of the TPN bag labels for expiration date, patient name, and patient date of birth; adding medications to the TPN infusion bag (eg, multivitamins, insulin); priming the infusion tubing; flushing protocol of the central line; disconnecting at the completion of the infusion; and signs and symptoms of infection. Helping the patient and family establish a clean work environment is critical to infection prevention. Proper storage of equipment must be reviewed and when possible the use of a separate refrigerator for storage of PN should be encouraged. Over each of 3 consecutive home teaching visits, the patient and/or caregiver will progressively become more involved in the TPN infusion with the end goal of the patient and/or caregiver completing a full teach back. To ensure the correct infusion technique is maintained after the initial teaching visits, the patient and/or caregiver will be scheduled for nursing visits to demonstrate the infusion to the nurse 14 days after start of care and in 6-month intervals ongoing.

To standardize nurse education, encourage patient participation, and decrease deviation from established TPN administration techniques, each patient is provided with a series of TPN teaching posters with images of equipment and solution handling and written instructions. These standardized documents allow nurses to educate patients in the same consistent way while also allowing the patient/caregiver to be confident in each step of the procedure.

ESTABLISH A COMPREHENSIVE AND CONSISTENT MONITORING PLAN

Our advanced practice nurses spend time with the potential HPN patient to review important clinical symptoms to monitor when at home. The potential for dehydration

---

Box 2
Patient training bullet list

- In-hospital training includes
  - Managing the infusion pump
  - Spiking the HPN infusion system
  - Connecting and disconnecting the tubing
  - Communication links with HPN supplier

- Visits in the home after discharge for training include
  - Gathering needed supplies
  - Retraining on managing the infusion pump
  - Confirming the appropriate HPN solution by reviewing the label
  - Adding multivitamins and medications such as insulin
  - Connecting and disconnecting the tubing to the central vascular access device
  - Increasing comfort with the HPN procedures

in the HPN patient is significant, and patients should be instructed to report symptoms such as dizziness, changes in thirst, decreased urine output, or weight loss. Equally important is the patient's understanding and recognizing signs of a catheter-related infection. They should be instructed to call if they experience redness or drainage from the catheter exit site. However, bloodstream infections are not usually associated with any symptoms at the exit site, instead the patient will experience fever and chills. The fever is often associated with active infusion, resolving when the infusion stops. It is important to alert the patient of this possibility and reinforce the importance of calling the health care provider immediately with any fever occurrence.

Ongoing contact between the patient and the HPN team is a cornerstone for effective care. Because these complex patients may have many other providers and health issues beyond their HPN care, weekly telephone calls can be an efficient way to find out how the HPN is going while obtaining information on other health concerns. Home infusion nursing visits for catheter management and blood draw also can provide useful information about the patient's clinical stability. It is best practice to avoid using the CVAD to draw bloodwork in the HPN patient to reduce the risk of infection.[4] The results of blood tests (initially weekly until stable, then monthly, then quarterly) and the risks of bloodwork drawn from the CVAD versus a peripheral blood draw are also important for management and a point of discussion and teaching with the patient and caregiver.

Although our patient care is largely provided by telephone and in face-to-face office visits, patients in more isolated settings may benefit from the use of technology in a telemedicine approach. Telemedicine has been reported in HPN patients as a strategy to detect symptoms of depression,[7] to monitor antibiotic therapy,[8] to provide routine monitoring with reduced CLABSI rates,[9] and to provide linked small group emotional support and education as a strategy to reduce complications.[10]

The best patient outcomes are achieved when the patient's care is coordinated across multiple essential providers.

Communication is eased and consistency of service provided by the use of usual clinical collaborators. Communication is eased and consistency of service provided by the use of usual clinical collaborators. Our service often works with 2 gastroenterologists, one with expertise in nutrition-related gastrointestinal disorders such as SBS and the other with dysmotility, the 2 most common long-term challenges of patients on our service. We also work regularly with an infectious disease specialist.

A collaborative relationship with gastroenterologists is key to the successful management of patients requiring HPN resulting from impaired GI function in many respects. For patients with underlying disease such as SBS, inflammatory bowel disease and/or dysmotility, medical management of symptoms with the ultimate goal of restoring GI function is central to liberation from HPN. Whether gut function can be fully or partially restored via medical management of disease is indeed patient- and disease-dependent and thus, consultative input from a gastroenterologist can aid in providing patients and the care team with valuable prognostic information that can help determine the course PN treatment For example, the GI output in a patient with SBS can in many instances be minimized through the use of antisecretory, antispasmotic, antidiarrheal, and digestive enzyme therapies that can result in reduced volume and kcal needs via PN. Furthermore, if and when the aforementioned medical therapies are ineffective, some patients with SBS are treated with growth factors and require colonoscopic screening and surveillance for polyps. A gastroenterologist with nutrition expertise also can make recommendations regarding oral intake in appropriate patients. Gut disease–focused diets such as FODMAP, lactose-free, and low fiber may be warranted in specific patients. In addition, patients with severe metabolic illness and/or GI symptoms may develop food aversion as a result of food-induced symptoms or significant appetite reduction with PN. These patients can be treated medically with appetite stimulant drugs, which may enable increased oral intake and quality of life.

The medical director of our most common home infusion supplier is an infectious disease specialist who monitors patients for CLABSI. A medical consultant with expertise in quality improvement, infection control, and/or infectious diseases can work with the patients' primary clinical nutrition team to optimize and decrease the risk of CLABSI and their sequelae. The consultant can strategize with other members of the team to address emergent IV access issues in patients who will require long-term central venous access. The medical consultant can participate with members of the primary nursing and nutrition teams in periodic case conference sessions during which ideas are exchanged and brain storming regarding new strategies to optimize the catheter care and education are exchanged. The medical consultant can stay abreast of current data regarding methods to decrease blood stream infections including ongoing evaluation of various catheters components, antiseptic techniques, novel dressings, and lock-therapy solutions. The medical consultant can then present these options to the members of the care team as options in given patients.

In addition to quality improvement and infection control role, the medical consultant can help facilitate multidisciplinary discussions for medically and socially complex patients and serve as a consultant to the patient's providers in making decisions regarding medical and antibiotic therapies for patients and in site of care decisions. These efforts can help a care team keep a patient out of the hospital by facilitating novel outpatient treatment approaches.

QUALITY OF LIFE

Our HPN patients and their caregivers are only rarely health professionals themselves. As noted previously, they undergo training in the care of the catheter and the HPN procedures. However, they may lack confidence about the provision of such high-risk care even after their training, which may result in CLABSI or catheter breakage. In addition, several factors may negatively impact the quality of life of HPN patients, including decreased physical, psychological, and social function; drug dependency; sleep disturbance and frequent urination during the infusion; fear of therapy-related complications; inability to eat; and financial distress.[11–16] Although patients may report a reduction in their quality of life in the early days of HPN, many also go on to report improvement over time.

The reason the patient requires HPN also can factor into the patient's initial interpretation of his or her situation. When a catastrophic event results in the need for HPN, the patient may be unprepared to implement strategies to adjust his or her lifestyle. By contrast, other patients may view HPN as a welcome relief to alleviate severe GI symptoms and chronic malnutrition. Finally, patients with advanced cancers that require HPN may not see the therapy as a cure, but rather as a way to maintain energy needed to fulfill a particular goal. Clinicians transitioning patients home on HPN should appreciate each patient's unique situation in order to support their compliance with a complex therapy, and know when to direct patients to a local or national support group for additional support.

SUMMARY

Preparing the patient for HPN is a collaborative effort among many different clinicians. Identifying patients who will transition home with PN as early as possible allows for a thoughtful and safe approach. Communication regarding the HPN goals is critical to the patient's success, whether the requirement for PN is temporary or permanent. Management of these complex patients is best served by a multidisciplinary team with expertise in the area of nutrition support. Adherence to available guidelines that define best practice is imperative in all aspects of care for the patient on HPN.

REFERENCES

1. Mundi MS, Pattinson A, McMahon MT, et al. Prevalence of home parenteral and enteral nutrition in the United States. Nutr Clin Pract 2017;32(6):799–805.
2. Howard L. Home parenteral nutrition in patients with a cancer diagnosis. JPEN J Parenter Enteral Nutr 1992;16(6 Suppl):93S–9S.
3. Winkler MF, DiMaria-Ghalili RA, Guenter P, et al. Characteristics of a cohort of home parenteral nutrition patients at the time of enrollment in the Sustain Registry. JPEN J Parenter Enteral Nutr 2016;40(8):1140–9.
4. Buchman AL, Opilla M, Kwasny M, et al. Risk factors for the development of catheter-related bloodstream infections in patients receiving home parenteral nutrition. JPEN J Parenter Enteral Nutr 2014;38(6):744–9.
5. Buchman AL. Catheter-related bloodstream infections in home parenteral nutrition patients and catheter salvage. Am J Clin Nutr 2018;108(5):1154.
6. Kovacevich DS, Corrigan M, Ross VM, et al. American Society for Parenteral and Enteral Nutrition guidelines for the selection and care of central venous access devices for adult home parenteral nutrition administration. JPEN J Parenter Enteral Nutr 2019;43(1):15–31.
7. Adams N, Hamilton N, Nelson EL, et al. Using telemedicine to identify depressive symptomatology rating scale in a home parenteral nutrition population. J Technol Behav Sci 2017;2(3–4):129–39.
8. Tan SJ, Ingram PR, Rothnie AJ, et al. Successful outpatient parenteral antibiotic therapy delivery via telemedicine. J Antimicrob Chemother 2017;72(10):2898–901.
9. Raphael BP, Schumann C, Garrlty-Gentille S, et al. Virtual telemedicine visits in pediatric home parenteral nutrition patients: a quality improvement initiative. Telemed J E Health 2019;25(1):60–5.
10. Nelson EL, Yadrich DM, Thompson N, et al. Telemedicine support groups for home parenteral nutrition users. Nutr Clin Pract 2017;32(6):789–98.
11. Winkler MF. Quality of life in adult home parenteral nutrition patients. JPEN J Parenter Enteral Nutr 2005;29(3):162–70.
12. Baxter JP, Fayers PM, McKinlay AW. A review of the quality of life of adult patients treated with long-term parenteral nutrition. Clin Nutr 2006;25(4):543–53.
13. Roskott AM, Huisman-de Waal G, Wanten GJ, et al. Screening for psychosocial distress in patients with long-term home parenteral nutrition. Clin Nutr 2013;32(3):396–403.
14. Silver HJ. The lived experience of home total parenteral nutrition: an online qualitative inquiry with adults, children, and mothers. Nutr Clin Pract 2004;19(3):297–304.
15. Aeberhard C, Leuenberger M, Joray M, et al. Management of home parenteral nutrition: a prospective multicenter observational study. Ann Nutr Metab 2015;67(4):210–7.
16. Winkler MF, Smith CE. Clinical, social, and economic impacts of home parenteral nutrition dependence in short bowel syndrome. JPEN J Parenter Enteral Nutr 2014;38(1 Suppl):32S–7S.

Etiology and Medical Management of Pediatric Intestinal Failure

Ethan A. Mezoff, MD[a],*, Conrad R. Cole, MD[b],
Valeria C. Cohran, MD[c]

KEYWORDS

- Pediatric intestinal failure • Short bowel syndrome • Parenteral nutrition

KEY POINTS

- Pediatric intestinal failure is a morbid and costly condition, the result of heterogeneous orphan diseases and surgical anatomies.
- Care of the child with intestinal failure seeks to achieve enteral autonomy in those capable and mitigate associated comorbidity in all.
- Multidisciplinary intestinal rehabilitation teams have driven improvement in outcomes in recent decades.
- Although long-term effectiveness has not yet been conclusively shown, new therapeutics and approaches to care brighten the future of care in children.

DEFINING INTESTINAL FAILURE

Pediatric intestinal failure (IF) occurs when gut digestive and absorptive function is insufficient to meet the growing body's fluid, electrolyte, and nutrient requirements.[1] A discrete, unambiguous, and broadly accepted definition has been elusive, with reports indicating a diagnosis of IF when an infant or child requires parenteral nutrition (PN) anywhere from 42 to 90 days, with or without qualifying statements of residual bowel length or pathology.[2–4] The infrequency with which this condition occurs and

Disclosures: The authors have nothing to disclose.
[a] Division of Gastroenterology, Hepatology and Nutrition, The Ohio State University College of Medicine, Center for Intestinal Rehabilitation and Nutrition Support, Nationwide Children's Hospital, 700 Children's Drive, Columbus, OH 43205, USA; [b] Division of Gastroenterology, Hepatology and Nutrition, University of Cincinnati College of Medicine, Cincinnati Children's Hospital Medical Center, 3333 Burnet Avenue, Cincinnati, OH 45229, USA; [c] Division of Gastroenterology, Hepatology and Nutrition, Feinberg School of Medicine, Northwestern University, The Ann & Robert H. Lurie Children's Hospital of Chicago, 225 East Chicago Box 65, Chicago, IL 60611, USA
* Corresponding author.
E-mail address: Ethan.Mezoff@nationwidechildrens.org

Gastroenterol Clin N Am 48 (2019) 483–498
https://doi.org/10.1016/j.gtc.2019.08.003
0889-8553/19/© 2019 Elsevier Inc. All rights reserved.

the heterogeneity of the population has further limited the depth and breadth of prospective evaluation and study of natural history of the condition.

CLASSIFICATION

The true incidence and prevalence of IF in North America are not known; however, a recent report of the prevalence in Italy estimated 14 cases per million inhabitants.[5] Primary classification of the etiologies comprising IF include short bowel syndrome (SBS), dysmotility, and mucosal enteropathy. Abdominal wall defects may be considered a fourth classification, because these patients may have features of both a decrease in gut length and primary dysmotility. SBS, resulting from loss of absorptive surface area, is the most common cause of IF with a population-based estimate of IF/SBS incidence in North America of 24.5 cases per 100,000 live births.[2] In 2012, Squires and colleagues,[4] reported the diagnostic composition of a cohort of 272 pediatric IF patients across 14 North American sites (**Table 1**).

ADAPTATION

After massive bowel resection, remnant bowel adapts to this loss of absorptive and digestive capacity through a process characterized in animal models by villus elongation and crypt deepening.[6] The process of adaptation can begin 24 hours after bowel resection and go on for years.[4,7] Adaptation ultimately facilitates the weaning of PN and thus has been a predominant focus of scientific study.

Many mediators of the adaptive response have been described. The presence and type of intraluminal nutrients are known to be important. Mucosal atrophy is observed in the absence of enteral nutrition and specific components and types, such as longer chain fats or human milk stimulate a greater adaptive response.[8–10] Indeed, we have shown the prebiotic human milk oligosaccharide 2'-fucosyllactose may be beneficial, providing additional evidence for the role of gut flora.[11,12] Humoral factors, a potential therapeutic target, have long been known to contribute to the adaptive response, including epidermal growth factor, glucagon-like peptide 2, and insulin-like growth factor.[13–15] Endogenous pancreaticobiliary secretions are also important.[16]

Remnant bowel anatomy, after resection, is predictive of the rate of adaptation and likelihood of achieving enteral autonomy. Residual small bowel length is consistently found to be a primary predictor of the duration of PN requirement and several nomograms have been published to predict likelihood of PN weaning by this measure (**Fig. 1**).[3,9,17] Preservation of the ileocecal valve, considered a brake on nutrient and fluid transit, and remnant colon independent of the ileocecal valve may be associated with the ability to achieve enteral autonomy.[3,9,18–21] The use of human milk or an amino acid-based formula, etiology of IF, and percentage of total calories received enterally in the weeks after surgery are also important.[3,9,18] Although these factors are helpful when discussing what the future may hold with the family of a newly diagnosed infant, the impact of attentive management throughout the routine care of the patient cannot be overstated.

PARENTERAL NUTRITION

PN, conceived more than 50 years ago, is a lifesaving, complex, and sterile cocktail of micronutrients and macronutrients delivered directly to venous circulation.[22] Dextrose is the primary carbohydrate source. Blood glucose is assessed periodically and the glucose infusion rate is kept below center standards, often at 15 mg/kg/min. A decrease in PN infusion hours is desirable for hepatoprotection

Table 1
Disease entities resulting in SBS

Author, Years	Number	Years	NEC	Gastroschisis	Intestinal Atresia	Volvulus	Combination	Hirschsprung's Disease	Other
Columb et al,[57] 2000	230	1980–1999	48 (16%)	48 (16%)	72 (24%)	NR	NR	39 (13%)	134 (44%)
Demeheri et al,[96] 2015	171	1988–2013	82 (43.9%)	42 (22.5%)	40 (21.4%)	34 (18.2%)	NR	NR	26 (13.9%)
Nucci et al,[97] 2008	389	1996–2006	74 (19%)	78 (20%)	47 (12%)	58 (15%)	NR	31 (8%)	26 (10.1%)
Squires et al,[4] 2012	272	2000–2007	71 (26%)	44 (16%)	27 (10%)	24 (9%)	46 (17%)	111 (4%)	48 (18%)
Fullerton et al,[98] 2016	313	2002–2014	95 (30%)	72 (23%)	52 (17%)	33 (11%)	NR	NR	22 (7%)

Abbreviation: NR, not reported.
Adapted from Cohran VC, Prozialeck JD, Cole CR. Redefining short bowel syndrome in the 21st century. Pediatr Res. 2017;81(4):540-549; with permission.

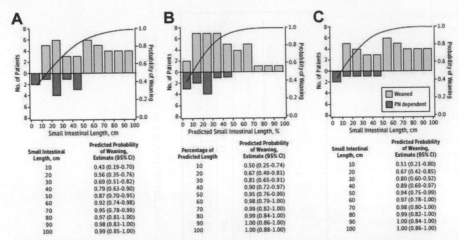

Fig. 1. Nomogram depicting theoretic relationship between the probability of weaning from PN. (*A*) Predicted probability based on small intestinal length. (*B*) Predicted probability based on percentage of predicted small intestinal length. (*C*) Predicted probability based on small intestinal length excluding patients who underwent bowel-lengthening procedures. The curved black line indicates predicted probability. Patients who died (n = 8) or underwent transplant (n = 4) were excluded. CI, confidence interval. (*From* Fallon EM, Mitchell PD, Nehra D, et al. Neonates with short bowel syndrome: an optimistic future for parenteral nutrition independence. JAMA Surg. 2014;149(7):663-670; with permission.)

and quality of life, but must be balanced against escalations in the glucose infusion rate and the responsiveness of insulin secretion after abrupt cessation; a 30- to 120-minute taper period is often used to prevent rebound hypoglycemia. Several protein solutions are available with differing essential and nonessential amino acid content, as well as the ratio of branched to aromatic chain amino acids. The traditional lipid source is derived from soy oil, however, new fat emulsions including olive, fish, and/or medium chain triglyceride oils are available. Lipid dosing balances potential hypertriglyceridemia with essential fatty acid deficiency, determined using the Holman index (triene/tetraene ratio) and levels of mead, linolenic, linoleic and arachidonic acid, as well as IF-specific comorbidities discussed elsewhere in this article.[23,24]

ENTERAL NUTRITION

The optimal enteral nutrition source, method and schedule of delivery, and advancement strategy are debated among experts and individually tailored in the course of care, although some general concepts are agreed upon. A key stimulus of adaptation, enteral nutrition should be introduced as soon as possible after bowel resection.[25] Human milk is the preferred choice and contains antimicrobial factors, prebiotic milk oligosaccharides, and growth hormones. When not available, an amino acid formula is the next choice for infants; both entities are associated with a shorter duration of PN use.[9] Children and adolescents may receive standard or blenderized polymeric formula supplementation. Early oral feeding protects from long-term oral aversion through stimulation and maintenance of oral skills, but does not always permit optimal advancement. Enteral tubes are commonly used and gastric feedings are preferred over jejunal to promote gastric and pancreatic secretion, use the complete gut surface, and facilitate skeletal motor development by minimizing continuous feedings during waking hours. We tailor feeding mode and route to the individual, often electing for continuous feedings overnight and bolus feedings through the day. The strategy for advancement balances both the need to consistently challenge remnant bowel for the purposes of stimulating adaptation and minimizing the development of comorbidity, over the avoidance of fluid and electrolyte deviations and growth failure associated with intolerance and malabsorption.

SYMPTOMATOLOGY AND MEDICATION MANAGEMENT

Infants or children with IF are at risk for a number of nonspecific complaints related to remnant bowel function, often requiring empiric drug trials with confounded evidence of improvement or ineffectiveness.

- Bowel dysmotility disorders are relatively common and treated with prokinetic agents such as erythromycin, amoxicillin–clavulanic acid, and octreotide.
- Liquid stools can be addressed with antimotility agents (eg, loperamide, clonidine, and other opioid agonists), antisecretory agents (eg, octreotide, proton pump inhibitors), and formula additives (eg, pectin or other sources of soluble fiber such as green beans).
  - o Elevated or liquid stoma output should first prompt assessment for mechanical, ischemic, or infectious problems.
- Microbial overgrowth of oropharyngeal and colonic flora may be indicated with reductions in nutrient absorption associated with flatulence and a decline in stool consistency. D-Lactic academia or cobalamin (B_{12}) deficiency may then occur. Aspiration and quantitative culture of proximal bowel contents is considered the gold standard for diagnosis ($>10^5$ colony-forming units), but invasiveness, cost, and reliability limit use. Treatment is generally empiric but important because overgrowth has been shown to increase the risk for bloodstream infection and prolong the duration of PN.[26,27] Although decreases in acid suppression and the dietary composition of simple sugars are important considerations, the mainstay of treatment is cycling of antimicrobials directed at anaerobic and gram-negative organisms.[28]

Prudence and caution are advocated, as well as a clear-eyed assessment of effectiveness, to avoid polypharmacy.

CENTRAL LINE COMPLICATIONS

Central venous access is necessary to sustain life in children with IF, but is a substantial source of infectious and thrombotic risk, interrelated and attributed to daily use and duration of need. As such, placement and maintenance requires thoughtful attention at the patient and program level. Central venous catheters are placed to the cavoatrial junction, conventionally through neck, arm, or subclavian veins. Peripherally inserted or tunneled, cuffed catheters with the smallest diameter and fewest lumens are preferred to decrease thrombotic and infectious complications.[29,30] Thrombosis from venous injury is a potential and concerning complication in many patients. Early recognition and intervention are necessary for preservation of venous access, although methods of late salvage, recanalization, and alternative site placements have been described.[31,32]

In addition to thrombotic complications, patients with central venous catheters are at increased risk for infection at the insertion site and blood stream. Conflicting needs to remove the infection source and to decrease the risk of thrombus formation from line removal and replacement must be balanced and generally result in removal only in the setting of clinical instability or failure to achieve blood sterility after 3 days of appropriate therapy.[33] Antibiotic-impregnated catheters and antibiotic lock solutions have been shown to decrease the risk of infection, but a theoretic risk of antibiotic resistance has limited use.[34,35] Ethanol is a broad spectrum antiseptic with the ability to penetrate biofilms, acting through disruption of cellular membranes, denaturation of microbial proteins, and cellular lysis.[36,37] Observational, single-center studies have decisively shown a decrease in catheter-related blood stream infection with prophylactic use at varying concentrations (70% is most common), and there may be less frequent catheter replacements, although repair rates may increase.[38,39]

INTESTINAL FAILURE-ASSOCIATED LIVER DISEASE

IF-associated liver disease (IFALD)—that is, reversible or irreversible hepatobiliary dysfunction associated with IF management—is a primary morbidity and one of the most important risk factors associated with mortality among infants with IF.[40,41] Criteria suggested for diagnosis have included the presence of serum direct or conjugated bilirubin levels of greater than 2 mg/dL among infants with IF and the absence of other causes of cholestasis.[42] Histopathologic examination reveals a picture of cholestasis with or without fibrosis or cirrhosis. Supporting findings may include evidence of portal hypertension or elevations in hepatic biochemical measures, although it should be noted that clinical and biochemical signs can be misleading and liver fibrosis may continue even years after PN discontinuation.[43] The incidence of IFALD among infants and children with IF is approximately 22% to 50%.[40,42,44]

Many host and microbial factors have been implicated in the development of IFALD. Intestinal obstruction and stasis, prematurity at birth, gut microbial community composition, and recurrent sepsis or hepatic Kupffer cell activation from circulating endotoxin have been proposed.[45–47] The route, type, and duration of nutrition source are also strongly associated with risk of IFALD; early trophic feeding promotes gut function and total duration of PN is strongly associated with IFALD risk.[40,48,49] All components of PN may promote cholestasis, however, most recent interest has been directed at intravenous lipid emulsions, specifically soy oil emulsion.[50,51] Proposed mechanisms of intravenous lipid emulsions toxicity include modulation of oxidative stress, through an abundance of ω-6 fatty acid precursors of the proinflammatory eicosanoids and a paucity of antioxidant α-tocopherol, as well as bile acid transporter inhibition by plant sterols.[45,46,52,53]

The prevention and treatment of IFALD seeks to address known and modifiable risks; however, high-quality evidence of effectiveness is lacking. Strategies to prevent blood stream infection, specifically the use of ethanol locks, are recommended.[45,54] The choleretic ursodeoxycholic acid, with possible benefit and without compelling evidence of harm, can be prescribed in the setting of elevated liver enzymes in children with or at risk for IFALD.[55] Intralipid emulsion dose reduction to 1 g/kg/d, suspension of lipid use, and reduction in number of days at greater than 2.5 g/kg/d may improve cholestasis and reduce risk for severe IFALD.[56,57] Relative to soy oil emulsion, fish oil emulsion contains no plant sterols and a more favorable ω-3:ω-6 fatty acid profile. A large body of observational, case-controlled, and, recently, randomized controlled studies have supported the use of fish oil emulsion preparation for the treatment of PN-associated cholestasis. A specific fish oil emulsion preparation is now approved by the US Food and Drug Administration for the treatment of IFALD.[52,58,59] A multicomponent emulsion containing 25% soy, 30% medium-chain triglyceride, 25% olive, and 15% fish oil has also been studied with positive result in children to limit the soy oil emulsion ω-6 oil load.[60,61] Unfortunately, conclusive data regarding the optimal dose and source of lipid emulsion in the prevention or treatment of IFALD, as well as impact on neurodevelopment, are lacking.[45,52]

MICRONUTRIENT DEFICIENCY

Vitamin and mineral absorption and sufficiency are important in the process of intestinal adaptation; however, postsurgical anatomy, length of bowel resected, and degree of malabsorption may cause micronutrient deficiency.[62] Indeed, a high prevalence of multiple micronutrient deficiencies occurs during and after the transition to enteral autonomy, including deficiencies of iron, copper, and fat-soluble vitamins.[63,64] These deficiencies lead to increased risk for infection, anemia, thrombosis, demyelinating disease, growth failure, metabolic bone disease, and other conditions. Although some center-specific variation exists, routine monitoring across 14 pediatric intestinal rehabilitation programs was recently described by Nucci and colleagues[65] (**Table 2**). Results of routine monitoring should be interpreted with caution because multiple confounders may be present, such as assay limitations and inflammation.[66,67] Achievement of sufficiency through enteral supplementation, although effective in many, may be challenging in the setting of malabsorption and decreased intestinal mass.

MORTALITY

Over the past 4 decades, overall survival with pediatric IF has improved dramatically and there has been a decline in intestinal transplantation rates. Survival spanning the last 2 decades of the 20th century was 70%, as reported from a tertiary care center.[68] A second report of this period confirmed a 2-year survival of 70%.[69] Reports of survival including the current decade are much more encouraging, with survival rates of 94% to 97%.[70-72] Risk of mortality seems to be greatest in the first 2 years after diagnosis and is related to IFALD, prematurity, race, and whether a child receives care at a center offering a multidisciplinary approach to management.[4,69,73-75]

Table 2
Laboratory tests routinely followed among pediatric patients with IF as reported in a practice survey of dietitians representing 14 intestinal rehabilitation programs across North America

	Panels	Vitamins	Trace Elements	Other
Frequency	Daily to monthly	Every 3–12 mo	Every 3–12 mo	Every 3–12 mo
Component	Comprehensive metabolic panel Basic metabolic panel Complete blood count	Serum retinol Retinol binding protein Red blood cell folate Vitamin B_{12} Methylmalonic acid Vitamin D Vitamin E	Serum copper Serum zinc Selenium Serum iron Total iron binding capacity Ferritin	Magnesium Phosphorous Serum triglycerides C-reactive protein Prothrombin time International normalized ratio Thyroid-stimulating hormone Serum citrulline Triene:tetraene ratio

Adapted from Nucci AM, Ellsworth K, Michalski A, et al, Section APIF. Survey of Nutrition Management Practices in Centers for Pediatric Intestinal Rehabilitation. *Nutr Clin Pract.* 2018;33(4):528-538; with permission.

INTESTINAL REHABILITATION PROGRAM

Few advancements in the care of children with IF have made as profound an impact as the implementation of a multidisciplinary team approach (**Fig. 2**).[74] It is recommended that intestinal rehabilitation programs be composed of, at a minimum, a gastroenterologist, surgeon, dietitian, and nurse providing dedicated care (**Table 3**).[76] Close collaboration with other providers is encouraged, including interventional radiologists, neonatologists, social workers, child psychologists, occupational and physical therapists, speech and feeding therapists, and child life specialists.[76] We have also found close collaboration with a committed fluoroscopist to be indispensable.[77]

ENDOSCOPY AND SURGICAL MANAGEMENT

Many nonspecific gastrointestinal signs and symptoms may occur in association with enteral intolerance, prolonging the wean from PN. Endoscopy offers the opportunity for visual inspection of the bowel, evaluation for dilation, acquisition of mucosal samples for histology and duodenal fluid for culture, and the performance of therapeutic maneuvers to achieve hemostasis, direct surgical resection, or dilate intestinal strictures.[78–80] Seventy percent of endoscopies among children with IF (or, among 89% of patients undergoing endoscopy) may yield abnormalities in bowel appearance, microbiology, or histopathology, such as the presence of eosinophilic gastrointestinal inflammation.[81,82] Recent work echoed the high prevalence of mucosal and anatomic

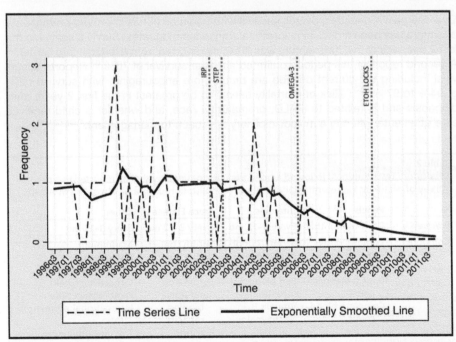

Fig. 2. The change in disease-specific mortality with treatment option expansion among pediatric patients with IF between 1996 and 2011 at a single study site. ETOH, ethanol; IRP, intestinal rehabilitation program; STEP, serial transverse enteroplasty. (*From* Oliveira C, de Silva NT, Stanojevic S, et al. Change of Outcomes in Pediatric Intestinal Failure: Use of Time-Series Analysis to Assess the Evolution of an Intestinal Rehabilitation Program. *J Am Coll Surg.* 2016;222(6):1180-1188 e1183; with permission.)

Table 3
Proposed members of pediatric intestinal rehabilitation programs

Professionals	Role and Services
Pediatric surgeons	Gastrointestinal surgery, central venous catheter procedures; inpatient and outpatient surgical management
Transplant surgeons	Assessment, surgery, immunosuppression
Pediatric gastroenterologists	Inpatient and outpatient medical management
Neonatologists	Initial inpatient management of premature and critically ill infants
Interventional radiologists	Central venous line management
Gastroenterology/PN nurses	Line and ostomy care, education
Pharmacists	Supervision, preparation of PN, drug–nutrient interactions
Registered dietitians	Nutritional monitoring and counseling, drug–nutrient interactions
Social workers	Access available resources; support
Physical, occupational, and speech therapists	Feeding, mobility and development
Child life specialists	Child and family support, education
Psychologists	Individual treatment and family support
Medical educators	Instruction on self-care

Adapted from Merritt RJ, Cohran V, Raphael BP, et al. Intestinal Rehabilitation Programs in the Management of Pediatric Intestinal Failure and Short Bowel Syndrome. *J Pediatr Gastroenterol Nutr.* 2017;65(5):588-596; with permission.

findings on endoscopy and, based on a high rate of unexpected findings unassociated with symptomatology, advocated endoscopy can be used as a screening tool among pediatric patients with IF.[83]

"Non-Transplant Surgery of Intestinal Failure" will be addressed by Kishore R. Iyer and colleague's article in this issue and "Indications for Intestinal Transplantation in Intestinal Failure" will be covered by Ivo G. Tzvetanov and colleague's article in this issue.

FUTURE DIRECTIONS AND MISCELLANEA

Despite the advances in management described, a small proportion of patients with IF will not experience sufficient intestinal adaptation for achievement of enteral autonomy. Nonpharmacologic bowel augmentation through the implantation of autologous, engineered tissue promises a novel method of increasing absorptive surface area without exposure to the immune mediated risks of allogeneic bowel transplantation or low donor availability, but remains in its infancy.[84]

Strategies to pharmacologically augment the adaptive process are a heavy focus of study in the field and promise a bright future. Of identified humoral factors influencing adaptation, an analog of glucagon-like peptide 2 (teduglutide) has reached clinical study.[85,86] Among adults with IF requiring PN 3 or more times per week for 12 months or more, significantly more experienced reductions of greater than 20% PN volume when treated with Teduglutide compared with placebo ($P<.01$), although there was large variation in response.[85] Factors positively associated with response in this phase III study of adults with IF and SBS included higher baseline parenteral volume needs and intestinal anatomy, specifically the presence of a jejunostomy or ileostomy compared with patients with all or part of the colon in continuity.[87] Results of the first

12-week, open-label study of pediatric IF related to SBS were encouraging, revealing a favorable short-term safety profile and trends toward PN decreases and enteral nutrition advancements.[88] A 24-week study has completed enrollment (ClincalTrials. gov, NCT02682381).

A substantial and immediate challenge to research in the field of intestinal rehabilitation stems from the nature of IF itself, an orphan disease process involving multiple etiologies, heterogeneous bowel anatomies, and lacking discrete and standardized definitions.[75] Management practices and referral patterns also vary greatly among intestinal rehabilitation programs and impact outcomes.[65] These population and center characteristics have greatly limited the ability to extract generalizable knowledge from single-center studies. In the past, multicenter study required time-consuming double documentation and a high activation energy for any single study. The recent, widespread use of the electronic health record offers the promise of tools to seamlessly integrate daily work and global study through sharable data capture that drives clinical documentation, quality improvement, collaborative clinical research, and safety.[89–92]

IF is a chronic, morbid, and costly disease, by some estimates exceeding US$200,000 dollars annually.[93,94] Emerging evidence also suggests the condition takes a toll on physical and emotional health, as well as social functioning of patients and families.[95] Medical management of this heterogeneous disease process seeks to achieve enteral autonomy in those capable and mitigate comorbid disease in all. Care has greatly improved in recent decades with coordinated and multidisciplinary care, new lipid preparations and dosing strategies, and efforts to reduce infectious events associated with the placement and maintenance of central venous catheters. The field will continue to advance, with a focus on developing new drugs or tissue engineering techniques to increase absorptive capacity, and new methods of collaborative study to integrate research and clinical care.

REFERENCES

1. Duggan CP, Jaksic T. Pediatric intestinal failure. N Engl J Med 2017;377(7): 666–75.
2. Wales PW, de Silva N, Kim J, et al. Neonatal short bowel syndrome: population-based estimates of incidence and mortality rates. J Pediatr Surg 2004;39(5): 690–5.
3. Sondheimer JM, Cadnapaphornchai M, Sontag M, et al. Predicting the duration of dependence on parenteral nutrition after neonatal intestinal resection. J Pediatr 1998;132(1):80–4.
4. Squires RH, Duggan C, Teitelbaum DH, et al. Natural history of pediatric intestinal failure: initial report from the Pediatric Intestinal Failure Consortium. J Pediatr 2012;161(4):723–8.e2.
5. Diamanti A, Capriati T, Gandullia P, et al. Pediatric chronic intestinal failure in Italy: report from the 2016 Survey on Behalf of Italian Society for Gastroenterology, Hepatology and Nutrition (SIGENP). Nutrients 2017;9(11) [pii:E1217].
6. Dekaney CM, Fong JJ, Rigby RJ, et al. Expansion of intestinal stem cells associated with long-term adaptation following ileocecal resection in mice. Am J Physiol Gastrointest Liver Physiol 2007;293(5):G1013–22.
7. Helmrath MA, VanderKolk WE, Can G, et al. Intestinal adaptation following massive small bowel resection in the mouse. J Am Coll Surg 1996;183(5):441–9.
8. Feldman EJ, Dowling RH, McNaughton J, et al. Effects of oral versus intravenous nutrition on intestinal adaptation after small bowel resection in the dog. Gastroenterology 1976;70(5 PT.1):712–9.

9. Andorsky DJ, Lund DP, Lillehei CW, et al. Nutritional and other postoperative management of neonates with short bowel syndrome correlates with clinical outcomes. J Pediatr 2001;139(1):27–33.

10. Choi PM, Sun RC, Guo J, et al. High-fat diet enhances villus growth during the adaptation response to massive proximal small bowel resection. J Gastrointest Surg 2014;18(2):286–94 [discussion: 294].

11. Mezoff EA, Hawkins JA, Ollberding NJ, et al. The human milk oligosaccharide 2'-fucosyllactose augments the adaptive response to extensive intestinal. Am J Physiol Gastrointest Liver Physiol 2016;310(6):G427–38.

12. Neelis E, de Koning B, Rings E, et al. The gut microbiome in patients with intestinal failure: current evidence and implications for clinical practice. JPEN J Parenter Enteral Nutr 2019;43(2):194–205.

13. Chaet MS, Arya G, Ziegler MM, et al. Epidermal growth factor enhances intestinal adaptation after massive small bowel resection. J Pediatr Surg 1994;29(8):1035–8 [discussion: 1038–9].

14. Tsai CH, Hill M, Asa SL, et al. Intestinal growth-promoting properties of glucagon-like peptide-2 in mice. Am J Physiol 1997;273(1 Pt 1):E77–84.

15. Knott AW, Juno RJ, Jarboe MD, et al. Smooth muscle overexpression of IGF-I induces a novel adaptive response to small bowel resection. Am J Physiol Gastrointest Liver Physiol 2004;287(3):G562–70.

16. Williamson RC, Bauer FL, Ross JS, et al. Contributions of bile and pancreatic juice to cell proliferation in ileal mucosa. Surgery 1978;83(5):570–6.

17. Fallon EM, Mitchell PD, Nehra D, et al. Neonates with short bowel syndrome: an optimistic future for parenteral nutrition independence. JAMA Surg 2014;149(7):663–70.

18. Khan FA, Squires RH, Litman HJ, et al. Predictors of enteral autonomy in children with intestinal failure: a multicenter cohort study. J Pediatr 2015;167(1):29–34.e1.

19. Spencer AU, Neaga A, West B, et al. Pediatric short bowel syndrome: redefining predictors of success. Ann Surg 2005;242(3):403–9 [discussion: 409–12].

20. Quiros-Tejeira RE, Ament ME, Reyen L, et al. Long-term parenteral nutritional support and intestinal adaptation in children with short bowel syndrome: a 25-year experience. J Pediatr 2004;145(2):157–63.

21. Nightingale JM, Lennard-Jones JE, Gertner DJ, et al. Colonic preservation reduces need for parenteral therapy, increases incidence of renal stones, but does not change high prevalence of gall stones in patients with a short bowel. Gut 1992;33(11):1493–7.

22. Dudrick SJ, Wilmore DW, Vars HM, et al. Long-term total parenteral nutrition with growth, development, and positive nitrogen balance. Surgery 1968;64(1):134–42.

23. Cober MP, Killu G, Brattain A, et al. Intravenous fat emulsions reduction for patients with parenteral nutrition-associated liver disease. J Pediatr 2012;160(3):421–7.

24. Holman RT. The ratio of trienoic: tetraenoic acids in tissue lipids as a measure of essential fatty acid requirement. J Nutr 1960;70(3):405–10.

25. Olieman JF, Penning C, Ijsselstijn H, et al. Enteral nutrition in children with short-bowel syndrome: current evidence and recommendations for the clinician. J Am Diet Assoc 2010;110(3):420–6.

26. Cole CR, Frem JC, Schmotzer B, et al. The rate of bloodstream infection is high in infants with short bowel syndrome: relationship with small bowel bacterial overgrowth, enteral feeding, and inflammatory and immune responses. J Pediatr 2010;156(6):941–7.e1.

27. Kaufman SS, Loseke CA, Lupo JV, et al. Influence of bacterial overgrowth and intestinal inflammation on duration of parenteral nutrition in children with short bowel syndrome. J Pediatr 1997;131(3):356–61.

28. Malik BA, Xie YY, Wine E, et al. Diagnosis and pharmacological management of small intestinal bacterial overgrowth in children with intestinal failure. Can J Gastroenterol 2011;25(1):41–5.

29. Early TF, Gregory RT, Wheeler JR, et al. Increased infection rate in double-lumen versus single-lumen Hickman catheters in cancer patients. South Med J 1990; 83(1):34–6.

30. Spencer TR, Mahoney KJ. Reducing catheter-related thrombosis using a risk reduction tool centered on catheter to vessel ratio. J Thromb Thrombolysis 2017;44(4):427–34.

31. Denny DF Jr. Venous access salvage techniques. Tech Vasc Interv Radiol 2011; 14(4):225–32.

32. Sullivan PM, Merritt R, Pelayo JC, et al. Recanalization of occluded central veins in a parenteral nutrition-dependent child with no access. Pediatrics 2018; 141(Suppl 5):S416–20.

33. Mermel LA, Allon M, Bouza E, et al. Clinical practice guidelines for the diagnosis and management of intravascular catheter-related infection: 2009 Update by the Infectious Diseases Society of America. Clin Infect Dis 2009;49(1):1–45.

34. Gilbert RE, Mok Q, Dwan K, et al. Impregnated central venous catheters for prevention of bloodstream infection in children (the CATCH trial): a randomised controlled trial. Lancet 2016;387(10029):1732–42.

35. Snaterse M, Ruger W, Scholte Op Reimer WJ, et al. Antibiotic-based catheter lock solutions for prevention of catheter-related bloodstream infection: a systematic review of randomised controlled trials. J Hosp Infect 2010;75(1):1–11.

36. Donlan RM. Biofilm elimination on intravascular catheters: important considerations for the infectious disease practitioner. Clin Infect Dis 2011;52(8):1038–45.

37. McDonnell G, Russell AD. Antiseptics and disinfectants: activity, action, and resistance. Clin Microbiol Rev 1999;12(1):147–79.

38. Rahhal R, Abu-El-Haija MA, Fei L, et al. Systematic review and meta-analysis of the utilization of ethanol locks in pediatric patients with intestinal failure. JPEN J Parenter Enteral Nutr 2018;42(4):690–701.

39. Oliveira C, Nasr A, Brindle M, et al. Ethanol locks to prevent catheter-related bloodstream infections in parenteral nutrition: a meta-analysis. Pediatrics 2012; 129(2):318–29.

40. Pichler J, Horn V, Macdonald S, et al. Intestinal failure-associated liver disease in hospitalised children. Arch Dis Child 2012;97(3):211–4.

41. Kocoshis SA. Medical management of pediatric intestinal failure. Semin Pediatr Surg 2010;19(1):20–6.

42. Lauriti G, Zani A, Aufieri R, et al. Incidence, prevention, and treatment of parenteral nutrition-associated cholestasis and intestinal failure-associated liver disease in infants and children: a systematic review. JPEN J Parenter Enteral Nutr 2014;38(1):70–85.

43. Mutanen A, Lohi J, Heikkila P, et al. Persistent abnormal liver fibrosis after weaning off parenteral nutrition in pediatric intestinal failure. Hepatology 2013;58(2): 729–38.

44. Cavicchi M, Beau P, Crenn P, et al. Prevalence of liver disease and contributing factors in patients receiving home parenteral nutrition for permanent intestinal failure. Ann Intern Med 2000;132(7):525–32.

45. Lacaille F, Gupte G, Colomb V, et al. Intestinal failure-associated liver disease: a position paper of the ESPGHAN Working Group of Intestinal Failure and Intestinal Transplantation. J Pediatr Gastroenterol Nutr 2015;60(2):272–83.

46. Lee WS, Sokol RJ. Intestinal microbiota, lipids, and the pathogenesis of intestinal failure-associated liver disease. J Pediatr 2015;167(3):519–26.

47. Korpela K, Mutanen A, Salonen A, et al. Intestinal microbiota signatures associated with histological liver steatosis in pediatric-onset intestinal failure. JPEN J Parenter Enteral Nutr 2017;41(2):238–48.

48. Zamir O, Nussbaum MS, Bhadra S, et al. Effect of enteral feeding on hepatic steatosis induced by total parenteral nutrition. JPEN J Parenter Enteral Nutr 1994;18(1):20–5.

49. Tyson JE, Kennedy KA. Trophic feedings for parenterally fed infants. Cochrane Database Syst Rev 2005;(3):CD000504.

50. Vileisis RA, Inwood RJ, Hunt CE. Prospective controlled study of parenteral nutrition-associated cholestatic jaundice: effect of protein intake. J Pediatr 1980;96(5):893–7.

51. Steinbach M, Clark RH, Kelleher AS, et al. Demographic and nutritional factors associated with prolonged cholestatic jaundice in the premature infant. J Perinatol 2008;28(2):129–35.

52. Hojsak I, Colomb V, Braegger C, et al, ESPGHAN Committee on Nutrition Position Paper. Intravenous lipid emulsions and risk of hepatotoxicity in infants and children: a systematic review and meta-analysis. J Pediatr Gastroenterol Nutr 2016;62(5):776–92.

53. Hukkinen M, Mutanen A, Nissinen M, et al. Parenteral plant sterols accumulate in the liver reflecting their increased serum levels and portal inflammation in children with intestinal failure. JPEN J Parenter Enteral Nutr 2017;41(6):1014–22.

54. Wales PW, Allen N, Worthington P, et al. A.S.P.E.N. clinical guidelines: support of pediatric patients with intestinal failure at risk of parenteral nutrition-associated liver disease. JPEN J Parenter Enteral Nutr 2014;38(5):538–57.

55. Arslanoglu S, Moro GE, Tauschel HD, et al. Ursodeoxycholic acid treatment in preterm infants: a pilot study for the prevention of cholestasis associated with total parenteral nutrition. J Pediatr Gastroenterol Nutr 2008;46(2):228–31.

56. Gura KM, Duggan CP, Collier SB, et al. Reversal of parenteral nutrition-associated liver disease in two infants with short bowel syndrome using parenteral fish oil: implications for future management. Pediatrics 2006;118(1): e197–201.

57. Colomb V, Jobert-Giraud A, Lacaille F, et al. Role of lipid emulsions in cholestasis associated with long-term parenteral nutrition in children. JPEN J Parenter Enteral Nutr 2000;24(6):345–50.

58. Lam HS, Tam YH, Poon TC, et al. A double-blind randomised controlled trial of fish oil-based versus soy-based lipid preparations in the treatment of infants with parenteral nutrition-associated cholestasis. Neonatology 2014;105(4):290–6.

59. Omegaven (fish oil triglycerides)[package insert]. Graz (Austria): Fresenius Kabi; 2018.

60. Diamond IR, Grant RC, Pencharz PB, et al. Preventing the progression of intestinal failure-associated liver disease in infants using a composite lipid emulsion: a pilot randomized controlled trial of SMOFlipid. JPEN J Parenter Enteral Nutr 2017; 41(5):866–77.

61. Goulet O, Antebi H, Wolf C, et al. A new intravenous fat emulsion containing soybean oil, medium-chain triglycerides, olive oil, and fish oil: a single-center, double-blind randomized study on efficacy and safety in pediatric patients

receiving home parenteral nutrition. JPEN J Parenter Enteral Nutr 2010;34(5): 485–95.

62. Mziray-Andrew CH, Sentongo TA. Nutritional deficiencies in intestinal failure. Pediatr Clin North Am 2009;56(5):1185–200.

63. Yang CF, Duro D, Zurakowski D, et al. High prevalence of multiple micronutrient deficiencies in children with intestinal failure: a longitudinal study. J Pediatr 2011; 159(1):39–44.e1.

64. Ubesie AC, Kocoshis SA, Mezoff AG, et al. Multiple micronutrient deficiencies among patients with intestinal failure during and after transition to enteral nutrition. J Pediatr 2013;163(6):1692–6.

65. Nucci AM, Ellsworth K, Michalski A, et al. Survey of nutrition management practices in centers for pediatric intestinal rehabilitation. Nutr Clin Pract 2018;33(4): 528–38.

66. Jimenez L, Stamm DA, Depaula B, et al. Is Serum methylmalonic acid a reliable biomarker of vitamin B12 status in children with short bowel syndrome: a case series. J Pediatr 2018;192:259–61.

67. Duncan A, Talwar D, McMillan DC, et al. Quantitative data on the magnitude of the systemic inflammatory response and its effect on micronutrient status based on plasma measurements. Am J Clin Nutr 2012;95(1):64–71.

68. Modi BP, Langer M, Ching YA, et al. Improved survival in a multidisciplinary short bowel syndrome program. J Pediatr Surg 2008;43(1):20–4.

69. Hess RA, Welch KB, Brown PI, et al. Survival outcomes of pediatric intestinal failure patients: analysis of factors contributing to improved survival over the past two decades. J Surg Res 2011;170(1):27–31.

70. Abi Nader E, Lambe C, Talbotec C, et al. Outcome of home parenteral nutrition in 251 children over a 14-y period: report of a single center. Am J Clin Nutr 2016; 103(5):1327–36.

71. Osakwe HI, Dragomir C, Nicolescu C, et al. The challenges of managing and following-up a case of short bowel in eastern Europe. Int J Surg Case Rep 2016;26:187–92.

72. Merras-Salmio L, Pakarinen MP. Refined multidisciplinary protocol-based approach to short bowel syndrome improves outcomes. J Pediatr Gastroenterol Nutr 2015;61(1):24–9.

73. Squires RH, Balint J, Horslen S, et al. Race affects outcome among infants with intestinal failure. J Pediatr Gastroenterol Nutr 2014;59(4):537–43.

74. Oliveira C, de Silva NT, Stanojevic S, et al. Change of outcomes in pediatric intestinal failure: use of time-series analysis to assess the evolution of an intestinal rehabilitation program. J Am Coll Surg 2016;222(6):1180–8.e3.

75. Stanger JD, Oliveira C, Blackmore C, et al. The impact of multi-disciplinary intestinal rehabilitation programs on the outcome of pediatric patients with intestinal failure: a systematic review and meta-analysis. J Pediatr Surg 2013;48(5):983–92.

76. Merritt RJ, Cohran V, Raphael BP, et al. Intestinal rehabilitation programs in the management of pediatric intestinal failure and short bowel syndrome. J Pediatr Gastroenterol Nutr 2017;65(5):588–96.

77. Lodwick D, Dienhart M, Ambeba E, et al. Accuracy of radiographic estimation of small bowel dimensions in pediatric patients with short bowel syndrome. J Pediatr Surg 2016;51(6):953–6.

78. Fusaro F, Tambucci R, Romeo E, et al. Anastomotic ulcers in short bowel syndrome: new suggestions from a multidisciplinary approach. J Pediatr Surg 2018;53(3):483–8.

79. Belza C, Fitzgerald K, Amaral J, et al. Use of balloon dilatation for management of postoperative intestinal strictures in children with short bowel syndrome. J Pediatr Surg 2017;52(5):760–3.

80. Bass LM, Zimont J, Prozialeck J, et al. Intestinal anastomotic ulcers in children with short bowel syndrome and anemia detected by capsule endoscopy. J Pediatr Gastroenterol Nutr 2015;61(2):215–9.

81. Stamm DA, Hait E, Litman HJ, et al. High prevalence of eosinophilic gastrointestinal disease in children with intestinal failure. J Pediatr Gastroenterol Nutr 2016; 63(3):336–9.

82. Ching YA, Modi BP, Jaksic T, et al. High diagnostic yield of gastrointestinal endoscopy in children with intestinal failure. J Pediatr Surg 2008;43(5):906–10.

83. Busch A, Sturm E. Screening endoscopy contributes to relevant modifications of therapeutic regimen in children with intestinal failure. J Pediatr Gastroenterol Nutr 2018;67(4):478–82.

84. Martin LY, Ladd MR, Werts A, et al. Tissue engineering for the treatment of short bowel syndrome in children. Pediatr Res 2018;83(1–2):249–57.

85. Jeppesen PB, Pertkiewicz M, Messing B, et al. Teduglutide reduces need for parenteral support among patients with short bowel syndrome with intestinal failure. Gastroenterology 2012;143(6):1473–81.e3.

86. Jeppesen PB, Sanguinetti EL, Buchman A, et al. Teduglutide (ALX-0600), a dipeptidyl peptidase IV resistant glucagon-like peptide 2 analogue, improves intestinal function in short bowel syndrome patients. Gut 2005;54(9):1224–31.

87. Jeppesen PB, Gabe SM, Seidner DL, et al. Factors associated with response to teduglutide in patients with short-bowel syndrome and intestinal failure. Gastroenterology 2018;154(4):874–85.

88. Carter BA, Cohran VC, Cole CR, et al. Outcomes from a 12-week, open-label, multicenter clinical trial of teduglutide in pediatric short bowel syndrome. J Pediatr 2017;181:102–11.e5.

89. Vanek VW, Ayers P, Kraft M, et al. A call to action for optimizing the electronic health record in the parenteral nutrition workflow. Nutr Clin Pract 2018;33(5): e1–21.

90. Noritz G, Boggs A, Lowes LP, et al. "Learn from every patient": how a learning health system can improve patient care. Pediatr Qual Saf 2018;3(5):e100.

91. Ramsey LB, Mizuno T, Vinks AA, et al. Learning health systems as facilitators of precision medicine. Clin Pharmacol Ther 2017;101(3):359–67.

92. Smith MD, Institute of Medicine (U.S.), Committee on the Learning Health Care System in America. Best care at lower cost : the path to continuously learning health care in America. Washington, DC: National Academies Press; 2013.

93. Kosar C, Steinberg K, de Silva N, et al. Cost of ambulatory care for the pediatric intestinal failure patient: one-year follow-up after primary discharge. J Pediatr Surg 2016;51(5):798–803.

94. Spencer AU, Kovacevich D, McKinney-Barnett M, et al. Pediatric short-bowel syndrome: the cost of comprehensive care. Am J Clin Nutr 2008;88(6):1552–9.

95. Hukkinen M, Merras-Salmio L, Pakarinen MP. Health-related quality of life and neurodevelopmental outcomes among children with intestinal failure. Semin Pediatr Surg 2018;27(4):273–9.

96. Demehri FR, Stephens L, Herrman E, et al. Enteral autonomy in pediatric short bowel syndrome: predictive factors one year after diagnosis. J Pediatr Surg 2015;50(1):131–5.

97. Nucci A, Burns RC, Armah T, et al. Interdisciplinary management of pediatric intestinal failure: a 10-year review of rehabilitation and transplantation. J Gastrointest Surg 2008;12(3):429–35 [discussion: 435–6].
98. Fullerton BS, Sparks EA, Hall AM, et al. Enteral autonomy, cirrhosis, and long term transplant-free survival in pediatric intestinal failure patients. J Pediatr Surg 2016; 51(1):96–100.

Predictors of Intestinal Adaptation in Children

Robert S. Venick, MD

KEYWORDS

- Enteral autonomy • Intestinal adaptation • Parenteral nutrition • Predictors
- Short-bowel syndrome

KEY POINTS

- Intestinal adaptation is a process that starts after intestinal resection, and is characterized by structural and functional changes that compensate for the loss of intestinal mucosal surface area and help increase absorptive capacity of the remnant bowel.
- Knowledge in pediatric intestinal rehabilitation is based mostly on relatively small single-center reports with limited multicenter consortium activity.
- Predictors of intestinal adaptation in children with intestinal failure include greater length of remnant small bowel, preservation of the ileocecal valve and colon, gastrointestinal continuity, diagnosis of necrotizing enterocolitis, enteral nutrition provided by breast milk or elemental formula, absence of complications including intestinal failure–associated liver disease and central line–associated blood stream infections and care received at a multidisciplinary intestinal rehabilitation program.

INTRODUCTION

Intestinal failure in pediatrics is defined as the inability of the small bowel to adequately absorb fluids, electrolytes, and nutrients that are required to support normal growth and development.[1,2] In children, short-bowel syndrome (SBS) accounts for two-thirds of the cases of intestinal failure, and motility disorders and congenital mucosal diarrheal disorders account for the remaining one-third.[3] Children with SBS are supported primarily by parenteral nutrition (PN), which has been the single-most important therapy contributing to their improved prognosis. Before the introduction of PN in the late 1960s, more than half of the children with SBS succumbed to complications of malnutrition, dehydration, and infection.[4,5] PN paved the way over the ensuing 50 years for significant improvements in the care and outcomes of pediatric SBS. In

Disclosure Statement: R.S. Venick has served as a site principal investigator for pediatric teduglutide trials (Gattex Shire Pharmaceuticals, Takeda Pharmaceuticals). No conflicts of interest to disclose.
Division of Pediatric GI, Hepatology and Nutrition, David Geffen School of Medicine, UCLA, Mattel Children's Hospital UCLA, Box 951752, Los Angeles, CA 90095, USA
E-mail address: Rvenick@mednet.ucla.edu

the current era, more than 90% of children with SBS who are cared for at experienced intestinal rehabilitation programs (IRPs) are expected to survive, and roughly 60% to 70% are expected to undergo intestinal adaptation and achieve full enteral autonomy.[6–11] This article focuses on the predictors of pediatric intestinal adaptation and discusses the pathophysiology and clinical management of children with SBS.

INTESTINAL ADAPTATION: DEFINITION, STRUCTURAL AND FUNCTIONAL CHANGES

The ultimate goal in the management of children with SBS is the achievement of independence from PN. The compensatory process involved in reaching enteral autonomy is intestinal adaptation. Clinically, it is demonstrated by the ability to wean PN and increase enteral nutrition (EN) over time while maintaining a child's nutritional status. Biologically, adaptation is best understood from animal models, in which it is known to start immediately after surgical resection of the bowel, and can continue for years.[12] Adaptation is characterized by structural and functional changes that compensate for the loss of intestinal mucosal surface area and help increase absorptive capacity of the remnant bowel.[13] Specific microscopic and morphologic changes include increases in villous height and crypt depth, myocyte and enterocyte proliferation, decrease in enterocyte apoptosis, and elongation and dilatation of the remnant small bowel.[14,15] These changes result in an increase in mucosal mass; enlargement in mucosal folds; and increase in muscle thickness, circumference, and length of the bowel. In the animal models of SBS, the initial phase of rapid cellular proliferation is associated with changes in expression of a variety of enterocyte-specific genes and microRNAs.[16–19]

Functional changes that occur with adaptation include changes in the expression of carrier-mediated transport, including upregulation of Na+/glucose cotransporters and Na+/H+ exchangers involved in absorption, as well as changes in the brush border membrane activity, fluidity, and permeability.[20–22] In addition, during adaptation there is a decrease in the intestinal transit rate, which affords the remnant small bowel more opportunity and time for nutrient absorption. Additional changes in the microbiome, barrier, and immune function of the bowel likely contribute to adaptation but are not yet as well described.[23]

TIMING OF INTESTINAL ADAPTATION

The timeframe over which intestinal adaptation occurs can be quite variable, with the most progress typically seen in the first few years following intestinal resection.[24] Within 24 months after resection, independence from PN has been reported in 43% to 84% of children with a history of intestinal failure.[7–9] Adaptation can last throughout childhood, as would be predicted by the natural linear growth of the intestinal tract during this period.

PROGNOSTIC FACTORS AND TIMING OF ADAPTATION IN SHORT-BOWEL SYNDROME

The likelihood of reaching enteral autonomy depends on the severity of gastrointestinal compromise and the absorptive capacity of the remnant bowel. Many studies have aimed to determine factors that make children with SBS more likely to depend on long-term PN versus develop enteral autonomy. Most of these reports are single-center, retrospective in nature, and composed of a relatively small number of children spanning over a prolonged period with variable endpoints and analyses (Table 1).[10,11,25–35] Factors that stand out from these studies include greater length

Table 1
Predictors of pediatric intestinal adaptation from single-center and multicenter analysis

Site	Time Period	No. of Children with SBS	Adaptation Rate, %	Predictors of Adaptation
Los Angeles, CA[27]	1975–2000	78	77	Small bowel length >15 cm, intact ICV, >50% of colon, GI continuity, fewer CLABSIs
Paris, France[26]	1975–1991	87	89	Small bowel length >40 cm, intact ICV
Boston, MA[10]	1986–1998	30	67	Small bowel length, enteral feeding with breast milk or elemental formula
Pittsburgh PA[29]	1996–2006	237	N/A	Small bowel length, lower initial total bilirubin at referral
Ann Arbor, MI[30]	1997–2003	80	64	Small bowel length >10% of expected, intact ICV
Toronto, CA[11]	1997–2001	40	63	Small bowel length >50% of expected, GI continuity
Boston, MA[31]	1996–2006	54	67	Small bowel length, diagnosis of necrotizing enterocolitis
North American Multicenter Pediatric Intestinal Failure Consortium[7]	2000–2004	272	43	Small bowel length, intact ICV, diagnosis of necrotizing enterocolitis, care provided at a nonintestinal transplant program

Abbreviations: CLABSI, central line–associated blood stream infection; GI, gastrointestinal; ICV, ileocecal valve.

of remnant small bowel, preservation of the ileocecal valve (ICV) and colon, gastrointestinal continuity, diagnosis of necrotizing enterocolitis as opposed to other causes of intestinal failure, EN provided from breast milk or elemental formula, avoidance of complications including intestinal failure–associated liver disease (IFALD) and central line–associated blood stream infections (CLABSIs), and care received at a multidisciplinary IRP.[6]

Length of Remnant Small Bowel

In 2012, the Pediatric Intestinal Failure Consortium (PIFCon), a North American consortium of 14 IRPs, reported in multivariate analysis of 272 children that a positive predictor of achieving intestinal adaptation was length of remnant small bowel >40 cm (odds ratio [OR] = 1.04).[3] As shown in **Table 1**, the length of remnant small bowel consistently stands out in large single-center reports as one of the most important predictors of reaching enteral autonomy, and is perhaps of maximal prognostic value in children when expressed as a percentage of length of small bowel expected for gestational age.[27,36]

The small intestine approximately doubles in length during the last trimester of an uncomplicated pregnancy, with children at 27 to 29 weeks of gestation having a mean of 100 cm, and those at 40 weeks of gestation having 150 to 200 cm of small bowel.[37] Given the marked increase in small bowel length that occurs late in gestation and the high frequency of prematurity in infants with necrotizing enterocolitis (NEC) and other congenital malformations, remnant small bowel length expressed as a fraction of expected for gestational age appears to be most useful.[36] Highlighting this, Spencer and colleagues[30] reported that a remnant small bowel length of less than 10% predicted was associated with a 5.7 times higher relative risk of mortality.

Ileocecal Valve and Colon

In a review article from the early 1970s, Wilmore[4] illustrated the importance that the ICV plays in intestinal adaptation, and also shed light on the importance of assessing the ICV in conjunction with the length of remnant small bowel and colon. This early report suggested that without an ICV, a jejunoileal segment of 38 cm was needed to reach enteral autonomy. Conversely, if the ICV was preserved, adaptation may occur with only 15 cm of remnant small bowel.[4] Subsequent single-center reports have also identified the presence of the ICV as an important prognostic factor[27] (see **Table 1**), and in the PIFCon report, the presence of an ICV (OR = 2.8) was also a multivariate positive predictor of intestinal adaptation.[3] Given that the ICV is rarely removed without some of the colon and terminal ileum, the exact significance of the ICV versus terminal ileum is difficult to judge.[27] Resection of the ileum generally reduces nutrient, fluid, and electrolyte absorption more so than resection of an equivalent length of proximal jejunum.[38,39] In contrast to the duodenum and jejunum, only the ileum actively reabsorbs bile acids, and if more than one-third of the ileum is lost, the compensatory increase in hepatic bile acid synthesis may not be able to keep pace with increased fecal bile acid loss.[13] In these cases, the proximal intestinal lumen bile salt concentration will be inadequate for efficient lipid emulsification, thereby contributing to steatorrhea. Furthermore, fat malabsorption increases colonic fluid loss, both because long-chain fatty acids hydroxylated by colonic bacteria stimulate colonocyte electrolyte and water secretion and because long-chain fatty acids are themselves impermeable to colonic epithelium, further increasing the total solute concentration in the colonic lumen.

Loss of ileum and ICV also adversely affects motility of the more proximal gut. Removal of the "ileal brake" accelerates gastric emptying of liquids and increases proximal small bowel motility directly, thereby shortening total intestinal transit time.[12,27] The result is a further reduction in contact time between luminal contents and the mucosal surface, adding to the aggregate reduction in nutrient, fluid, and electrolyte assimilation. Hormones normally secreted by the distal ileal mucosa, including peptide YY (PYY), and glucagon-like peptide 1 and 2 (GLP-1, GLP-2), also play important roles in SBS and intestinal adaptation.[40] In a single-center analysis of 78 children with SBS who required long-term PN, resection of 50% of the colon (P<.05) and the inability to re-establish intestinal continuity (P<.01) were negative predictors for reaching enteral autonomy.[27] In another series of 28 children who had less than 20 cm of small bowel, those with an intact colon that was in continuity were more likely to achieve nutritional autonomy.[41]

The colon plays an important role in fluid and electrolyte absorption as well as absorption of short-chain and medium-chain fatty acids. Specifically, starches that escape absorption in the small intestine and also soluble fibers are salvaged in the colon with fermentation to bioavailable short-chain fatty acids—primarily acetic, propionic, and butyric acid—by resident anaerobic bacteria.[42–47] Uptake of short-chain fatty acid molecules in the colon also creates an osmotic gradient that enhances water absorption, thereby limiting total fecal fluid loss.

Etiology of Short-Bowel Syndrome

The underlying cause of intestinal failure has often been suspected as affecting outcome. Gastroschisis, in particular those cases with associated intestinal atresia, has been reported as having a worse prognosis than other congenital malformations. This may be in part due to the associated gastrointestinal dysmotility frequently seen in infants with gastroschisis which presents another hurdle in the successful advancement of enteral feeds.[48–50]

In the PIFCon analysis, the diagnosis of necrotizing enterocolitis (OR = 2.4), compared with other causes of intestinal failure (IF), was a positive predictor for intestinal adaptation.[3,7] Indeed, infants with NEC were not only more likely to achieve enteral autonomy, but did so more rapidly even when, adjusted for remnant small bowel length, status of ICV, and institution where care was provided.[7] Although single-center analyses have not all reported a favorable association with NEC and intestinal adaptation,[51] it is possible that these analyses were hampered by small sample size, and/or high rate of associated morbidities of prematurity in infants with NEC.

The Role of Enteral Nutrition in Intestinal Adaptation

Intestinal adaptation is mediated by a variety of mechanical, humoral, and nutritional stimuli.[52,53] One of the best-established stimulants of adaptation is the presence of nutrients in the intestinal lumen, as mucosal hypoplasia will occur in the absence of enteral feeds.[4,24,37,54,55] Timely initiation of enteral feeding after small bowel resection has been reported to improve the rate of achieving enteral autonomy[56] Having said this, the evidence for the optimal type of EN in pediatric intestinal failure is limited and of poor quality, making guidelines in this area based more on clinical practice and experience than evidence.[57,58] In the PIFCon registry, only approximately 20% of patients received breast milk and 40 different types of formula were used, making it impossible to draw any meaningful conclusions regarding the optimal type of EN.[3,7]

For infants with SBS, breast milk is often recommended when available. Human milk contains growth factors (GLP-2, insulinlike growth factor-1, growth hormone, and interleukin-11), amino acids, immunoglobulins, and other immunologically important compounds that may promote intestinal adaptation.[10,59] When breast milk is unavailable, elemental (amino acid–based) formula is an alternative that has been touted, especially among North American centers, over peptide-based (protein hydrolysates) or intact protein formulas. In part this is because of a reduced tendency of elemental formulas to precipitate hypersensitivity reactions, and in part because of the belief that such formulas are more easily absorbed in SBS.[60,61] As such, Andorsky and colleagues[10] observed a shorter duration of PN for infants with SBS who received elemental formulas.

A paucity of data also exists with regard to the optimal mode (continuous vs bolus) and route of delivery of EN (oral vs nasogastric or gastrostomy tube vs post-pyloric) in children with SBS. In many IRPs, continuous gastric feeds are used in the early postoperative period following intestinal resection, as they may be better tolerated and less likely to be associated with reflux than bolus feeds.[6] This strategy allows for early maximal absorption of calories and fluids delivered into the gastrointestinal tract.[62–64] The delivery of continuous tube feeds, however, must be weighed against permitting some oral feeding in order to prevent oral aversion.[6] Some have also questioned whether continuous feeds predisposes children with SBS to bacterial translocation.[65] Advantages of oral or bolus feeds may include that they stimulate gastrointestinal hormonal surges (insulin, gastrin, and gastric inhibitory peptide), which may promote adaptation.[66] Bolus enteral feeds are regarded as most closely reproducing natural gastrointestinal physiology.[67] In many IRPs, it is not uncommon to use an approach that includes both continuous feeding at night and bolus feeding during the day.[6] In addition, the introduction of age-appropriate foods by mouth starting at 6 months of age, and the delivery of pureed foods via gastrostomy tube bolus are recently, increasingly popular strategies at many IRPs.

Avoidance of Parenteral Nutrition–Associated Complications

Although PN is most often life-sustaining for patients with SBS, long-term PN administration can be associated with its own potentially life-threatening complications that can hinder the adaptation process. Avoiding complications such as IFALD and CLABSIs is crucial in achieving enteral autonomy.

IFALD is defined biochemically by a rise in liver function tests (often serum total bilirubin >2.0 mg/dL) in patients with IF on PN in the absence of other causes. Clinically it can present with a spectrum of signs and symptoms ranging from hepatomegaly, jaundice, gallstones, and portal hypertension to end-stage liver disease. Histologic features of IFALD in children include variable portal and lobular inflammation, cholestasis, macrophage hyperplasia, and interlobular bile duct proliferation with varying degrees of portal and lobular fibrosis that may progress to cirrhosis.[68] The incidence of IFALD in the historical PIFCon cohort from 2000 to 2004 was 74%,[6] whereas a more recent systematic review of more than 20 studies reported the incidence at 30%.[69] Historically, 25% to 50% of patients with advanced IFALD who were unable to wean from PN went on to develop end-stage liver disease,[70] as demonstrated by 26% of the children in the PIFCon cohort requiring intestinal transplantation and 27% dying.[3] Historically, children with advanced IFALD have had worse probability of adaptation and survival.[3,6,27] Factors that contribute to IFALD include a paucity of EN, small intestinal bacterial overgrowth with bacterial translocation, CLABSIs and PN-associated factors including excessive PN calories, prolonged duration of PN infusion, and intravenous lipid dose and content.[71] Cholestasis in children with SBS contributes to malabsorption, which by nature is detrimental in reaching enteral autonomy.[6]

Strategies such as lipid minimization (1 g/kg per day), replacement of soy-bean lipid emulsions with fish oil (FO)-based or FO-inclusive emulsions (Omegaven or SMOF), which have higher Omega-3, higher Vitamin E content, and lower amounts of phytosterols, have helped significantly to reduce the prevalence of advanced IFALD over the past decade, simultaneously expanding the window of opportunity for intestinal adaptation.[72–77]

In children with SBS, the incidence and severity of IFALD is worsened by bacterial and fungal sepsis. CLABSIs in and of themselves have been shown by Belza and colleagues[78] in a regression analysis of a large single-center IRP to be a negative predictor of enteral autonomy with each septic episode per 1000 catheter days associated with a 5% decrease in odds ratio of adaptation. Subsequently, strategies that reduce risks of CLABSI for children with SBS on PN are crucial, as frequent CLABSIs can drive patients further away from intestinal adaptation.

CLABSIs account for a major source of morbidity in SBS. In pediatric patients with SBS, rates of infection have ranged between 1 and 6 per 1000 days of PN.[79,80] Strategies that have been advocated as important in lowering risks of CLABSIs for children with SBS on PN include identifying high-risk patients (ie, young children, with ostomies and gastrostomy tubes), avoiding femoral lines when at all possible, supporting quality improvement and continuing education programs for caregivers, and emphasizing the importance of meticulous hygiene and aseptic technique when accessing central venous catheters.[81]

Newer practical techniques used by some IRPs to lower CLABSI rates include the use of Biopatch and SwabCap. Routine use of antimicrobial or ethanol lock solutions during "off" periods of the PN cycle have been advocated either universally or for high-risk patients.[75,82] The routine use of ethanol locks has been shown in single-center studies to significantly reduce the rate of CLABSIs (University of Michigan, n = 15 children 8.0 ± 5.4 CLABSI/1000 catheter days before ethanol lock therapy vs 1.3 ± 3.0 after ethanol lock therapy, P<.01).[83] Some groups have shown a higher risk of CLABSIs in patients with SBS and small intestinal bacterial overgrowth (SIBO),[84] making strategies that reduce acid suppression, address dysmotility, and possibly use cyclic enteral antibiotics and probiotics worthwhile considerations to promote intestinal adaptation.

Intestinal Rehabilitation Programs

Significant progress in the outcomes of children with SBS has been reported from pediatric IRPs. Specifically, survival has climbed from 54% before 1972 to 94% in the modern era.[35] Along these same lines, adaptation rates have risen and intestinal transplantation rates began to decline worldwide in 2007, in large part because of improvements in the multidisciplinary management of children with intestinal failure.[85] Multidisciplinary teams at IRPs include pediatric gastroenterology, pediatric surgery, dietitians, clinical nurse specialists, feeding therapists, and social workers. IRPs provide continuity of care, with an emphasis on detailed patient and family education aimed at prevention, early recognition, and treatment of potential complications.[86] Single-center studies and a meta-analysis have described the important role of IRPs in achieving improved outcomes in this field.[35,87,88] For such reasons, IRPs have been endorsed by the North American Society for Pediatric Gastroenterology, Hepatology, and Nutrition.[86]

Emerging Biomarkers and Novel Therapies for Intestinal Adaptation

Citrulline, a nonessential amino acid produced by enterocytes in the small intestine, appears to vary in proportion to the length of small intestine or remnant enterocyte mass.[89] Plasma citrulline level has been used as a biomarker that may be helpful in predicting intestinal adaptation. Specifically, in small pediatric series (n = 24–27 children), citrulline concentrations >15 to 19 μmol/L seem to be indicative of children who will reach enteral autonomy.[89,90] Certainly larger, prospective studies are required to determine the utility of citrulline in this setting.

Pharmacotherapy with intestinotrophic hormones that help induce adaptation appear potentially promising for some particular patients. GLP-2 is one such hormone that is produced by L-cells of the ileum and cecum, and appears to enhance nutrient absorption by increasing crypt cell proliferation and survival, and decreasing gastrointestinal motility and secretions.[91] Endogenous GLP-2 has a relatively short half-life and is inactivated by the enzyme dipeptidyl dipeptidase. Teduglutide (Takeda) is a recombinant GLP-2 analogue with a single amino acid substitution that results in an extended half-life.[92] Teduglutide was approved by the US Food and Drug Administration for adults with SBS in 2012 after a series of studies showed increases in absorption, villous height, and crypt depth and decreases in PN needs.[93,94] A multicenter, randomized, open-label 12-week trial (n = 42 children) comparing teduglutide at 0.025 or 0.05 mg/kg per day with standard of care treatment demonstrated a trend toward a reduction in PN.[95] A 24-week (ClinicalTrials.gov number, NCT02682381) and pediatric extension trials are under way.

SUMMARY

The prognosis of children with IF has significantly improved over the past few decades such that 60% to 70% of children with SBS are expected to achieve enteral autonomy. Predictors of pediatric intestinal adaptation include greater length of remnant small bowel, preservation of the ICV and colon, gastrointestinal continuity, diagnosis of necrotizing enterocolitis, EN provided from breast milk or elemental formula, avoidance of IFALD and CLABSI, and care received at a multidisciplinary IRP. Potential novel therapies and predictors of intestinal adaptation contribute to the bright outlook for children with SBS.

REFERENCES

1. Goulet O, Ruemmele F, Lacaille F, et al. Irreversible intestinal failure. J Pediatr Gastroenterol Nutr 2004;38(3):250–69.
2. Kocoshis SA, Beath SV, Booth IW, et al, North American Society for Gastroenterology, Hepatology and Nutrition. Intestinal failure and small bowel transplantation, including clinical nutrition: Working Group report of the second World Congress of Pediatric Gastroenterology, Hepatology, and Nutrition. J Pediatr Gastroenterol Nutr 2004;39(Suppl 2):S655–61.
3. Squires RH, Duggan C, Teitelbaum DH, et al, Pediatric Intestinal Failure Consortium. Natural history of pediatric intestinal failure: initial report from the Pediatric Intestinal Failure Consortium. J Pediatr 2012;161(4):723–8.e2.
4. Wilmore DW. Factors correlating with a successful outcome following extensive intestinal resection in newborn infants. J Pediatr 1972;80(1):88–95.
5. Wilmore DW, Dudrick SJ. Growth and development of an infant receiving all nutrients exclusively by vein. JAMA 1968;203(10):860–4.
6. Duggan CP, Jaksic T. Pediatric intestinal failure. N Engl J Med 2017;377(7): 666–75.
7. Khan FA, Squires RH, Litman HJ, et al, Pediatric Intestinal Failure Consortium. Predictors of enteral autonomy in children with intestinal failure: a multicenter cohort study. J Pediatr 2015;167(1):29–34.e1.
8. Sigalet D, Boctor D, Brindle M, et al. Elements of successful intestinal rehabilitation. J Pediatr Surg 2011;46(1):150–6.
9. Torres C, Sudan D, Vanderhoof J, et al. Role of an intestinal rehabilitation program in the treatment of advanced intestinal failure. J Pediatr Gastroenterol Nutr 2007; 45(2):204–12.
10. Andorsky DJ, Lund DP, Lillehei CW, et al. Nutritional and other postoperative management of neonates with short bowel syndrome correlates with clinical outcomes. J Pediatr 2001;139:27–33.
11. Wales PW, de Silva N, Kim JH, et al. Neonatal short bowel syndrome: a cohort study. J Pediatr Surg 2005;40:755–62.
12. Tavakkolizadeh A, Whang EE. Understanding and augmenting human intestinal adaptation: a call for more clinical research. JPEN J Parenter Enteral Nutr 2002;26:251–5.
13. Buchman AL, Scolapio J, Fryer J. AGA technical review on short bowel syndrome and intestinal transplantation. Gastroenterology 2003;124:1111–34.
14. Welters CFM, Dejong CHC, Deutz NEP, et al. Intestinal adaptation in short bowel syndrome. ANZ J Surg 2002;72:229–36.
15. Scott RB, Sheehan A, Chin BC, et al. Hyperplasia of the muscularis propria in response to massive intestinal resection in rat. J Pediatr Gastroenterol Nutr 1995;21:399–409.
16. Juno RJ, Knott AW, Profitt SA, et al. Preventing enterocyte apoptosis after massive small bowel resection does not enhance adaptation of the intestinal mucosa. J Pediatr Surg 2004;39:907.

17. Stern LE, Erwin CR, Falcone RA, et al. cDNA microarray analysis of adapting bowel after intestinal resection. J Pediatr Surg 2001;36:190.
18. Erwin CR, Jarboe MD, Sartor MA, et al. Developmental characteristics of adapting mouse small intestine crypt cells. Gastroenterology 2006;130:1324.
19. Balakrishnan A, Stearns AT, Park PJ, et al. Upregulation of proapoptotic microRNA mir-125a after massive small bowel resection in rats. Ann Surg 2012;255:747.
20. Musch MW, Bookstein C, Rocha F, et al. Region-specific adaptation of apical Na/H exchangers after extensive proximal small bowel resection. Am J Physiol Gastrointest Liver Physiol 2002;283:G975–85.
21. Hines OJ, Bilchik AJ, Zinner MJ, et al. Adaptation of the Na+/glucose cotransporter following intestinal resection. J Surg Res 1994;57:22–7.
22. Thiesen A, Drozdowski L, Iordache C, et al. Adaptation following intestinal resection: mechanisms and signals. Best Pract Res Clin Gastroenterol 2003;17:981.
23. AU Joly F, Mayeur C, Bruneau A, et al. Drastic changes in fecal and mucosa-associated microbiota in adult patients with short bowel syndrome. Biochimie 2010;92(7):753–61.
24. Pironi L, Paganelli GM, Miglioli M, et al. Morphologic and cytoproliferative patterns of duodenal mucosa in two patients after long-term total parenteral nutrition: changes with oral refeeding and relation to intestinal resection. JPEN J Parenter Enteral Nutr 1994;18:351–4.
25. Dorney SF, Ament ME, Berquist WE, et al. Improved survival in very short small bowel of infancy with use of long-term parenteral nutrition. J Pediatr 1985;107:521–5.
26. Goulet O, Baglin-Gobet S, Talbotec C, et al. Outcome and long-term growth after extensive small bowel resection in the neonatal period: a survey of 87 children. Eur J Pediatr Surg 2005;15:95–101.
27. Quiros-Tejeira RE, Ament ME, Reyen L, et al. Long-term parenteral nutritional support and intestinal adaptation in children with short bowel syndrome: a 25-year experience. J Pediatr 2004;145:157–63.
28. Colomb V, Dabbas-Tyan M, Taupin P, et al. Long-term outcome of children receiving home parenteral nutrition: a 20-year single-center experience in 302 patients. J Pediatr Gastroenterol Nutr 2007;44:347–53.
29. Nucci A, Burns RC, Armah T, et al. Interdisciplinary management of pediatric intestinal failure: a 10-year review of rehabilitation and transplantation. J Gastrointest Surg 2008;12:429–35 [discussion: 35–6].
30. Spencer AU, Neaga A, West B, et al. Pediatric short bowel syndrome: redefining predictors of success. Ann Surg 2005;242:403–9 [discussion: 9–12].
31. Modi BP, Langer M, Ching YA, et al. Improved survival in a multidisciplinary short bowel syndrome program. J Pediatr Surg 2008;43:20–4.
32. Sudan D, DiBaise J, Torres C, et al. A multidisciplinary approach to the treatment of intestinal failure. J Gastrointest Surg 2005;9:165–76 [discussion: 76–7].
33. Sigalet D, Boctor D, Robertson M, et al. Improved outcomes in paediatric intestinal failure with aggressive prevention of liver disease. Eur J Pediatr Surg 2009; 19:348–53.
34. Javid PJ, Malone FR, Bittner R, et al. The optimal timing of referral to an intestinal failure program: the relationship between hyperbilirubinemia and mortality. J Pediatr Surg 2011;46:1052–6.
35. Fullerton BS, Sparks EA, Hall AM, et al. Enteral autonomy, cirrhosis, and long term transplant-free survival in pediatric intestinal failure patients. J Pediatr Surg 2016; 51:96–100.
36. Wales PW, Christison-Lagay ER. Short bowel syndrome: epidemiology and etiology. Semin Pediatr Surg 2010;19(1):3–9.

37. Struijs MC, Diamond IR, de Silva N, et al. Establishing norms for intestinal length in children. J Pediatr Surg 2009;44(5):933–8.
38. Sundaram A, Koutkia P, Apovian CM. Nutritional management of short bowel syndrome in adults. J Clin Gastroenterol 2002;34:207–20.
39. Jeppesen PB, Mortensen PB. Colonic digestion and absorption of energy from carbohydrates and medium-chain fat in small bowel failure. JPEN J Parenter Enteral Nutr 1999;23:S101–5.
40. Nightengale JMD, Kamm MA, van der Sijp JRM, et al. Gastrointestinal hormones in short bowel syndrome. Peptide YY may be the "colonic brake" to gastric emptying. Gut 1996;39:267–72.
41. Infantino BJ, Mercer DF, Hobson BD, et al. Successful rehabilitation in pediatric ultrashort small bowel syndrome. J Pediatr 2013;163:1361–6.
42. Olesen M, Gudmand-Høyer E, Holst JJ, et al. Importance of colonic bacterial fermentation in short bowel patients. Small intestinal malabsorption of easily digestible carbohydrate. Dig Dis Sci 1999;44:1914–23.
43. Royall D, Wolever TM, Jeejeebhoy KN. Evidence for colonic conservation of malabsorbed carbohydrate in short bowel syndrome. Am J Gastroenterol 1992;87:751–6.
44. Cummings JH. Colonic absorption: the importance of short chain fatty acids in man. Scand J Gastroenterol Suppl 1984;93:89–99.
45. Lifschitz CH, Carrazza FR, Feste AS, et al. In vivo study of colonic fermentation of carbohydrate in infants. J Pediatr Gastroenterol Nutr 1995;20:59–64.
46. Steed KP, Bohemen EK, Lamont GM, et al. Proximal colonic response and gastrointestinal transit after high and low fat meals. Dig Dis Sci 1993;38:1793–800.
47. Nordgaard I, Hansen BS, Mortensen PB. Importance of colonic support for energy absorption as small bowel failure proceeds. Am J Clin Nutr 1996;64:222–31.
48. Dicken BJ, Sergi C, Rescorla FJ, et al. Medical management of motility disorders in patients with intestinal failure: a focus on necrotizing enterocolitis, gastroschisis, and intestinal atresia. J Pediatr Surg 2011;46(8):1618–30.
49. Fullerton BS, Velazco CS, Sparks EA, et al. Contemporary outcomes of infants with gastroschisis in North America: a multicenter cohort study. J Pediatr 2017;188:192–7.
50. Sala D, Chomto S, Hill S. Long-term outcomes of short bowel syndrome requiring long-term/home intravenous nutrition compared in children with gastroschisis and those with volvulus. Transplant Proc 2010;42:5–8.
51. Georgeson K, Breaux C Jr. Outcome and intestinal adaptation in neonatal short-bowel syndrome. J Pediatr Surg 1992;27:344–50.
52. Chen G, Sun L, Yu M, et al. The Jagged-1/Notch-1/Hes-1 pathway is involved in intestinal adaptation in a massive small bowel resection rat model. Dig Dis Sci 2013;58:2478–86.
53. Rubin DC, Levin MS. Mechanisms of intestinal adaptation. Best Pract Res Clin Gastroenterol 2016;30:237–48.
54. DiBaise JK, Young RJ, Vanderhoof JA. Intestinal rehabilitation and the short bowel syndrome: part 1. Am J Gastroenterol 2004;99(7):1386.
55. Buchman AL, Moukarzel AA, Bhuta S. Parenteral nutrition is associated with intestinal morphologic and functional changes in humans. JPEN J Parenter Enteral Nutr 1995;19:453–60.
56. Sondheimer JM, Cadnapaphornchai M, Sontag M, et al. Predicting the duration of dependence on parenteral nutrition after neonatal intestinal resection. J Pediatr 1998;132:80–4.

57. Barclay AR, Beattie LM, Weaver LT, et al. Systematic review: medical and nutritional interventions for the management of intestinal failure and its resultant complications in children. Aliment Pharmacol Ther 2011;33(2):175–84.
58. Capriati T, Nobili V, Stronati L, et al. Enteral nutrition in pediatric intestinal failure: does initial feeding impact on intestinal adaptation? Expert Rev Gastroenterol Hepatol 2017;11(8):741–8.
59. Vanderhoof JA, Grandjean CJ, Kaufman SS, et al. Effect of high percentage medium-chain triglyceride diet on mucosal adaptation following massive bowel resection in rats. JPEN J Parenter Enteral Nutr 1984;8:685–9.
60. Bines J, Francis D, Hill D. Reducing parenteral requirement in children with short bowel syndrome: impact of an amino acid-based complete infant formula. J Pediatr Gastroenterol Nutr 1998;26:123–8.
61. De Greef E, Mahler T, Janssen A, et al. The influence of Neocate in paediatric short bowel syndrome on PN weaning. J Nutr Metab 2010;2010 [pii:297575].
62. Parker P, Stroop S, Greene H. A controlled comparison of continuous versus intermittent feeding in the treatment of infants with intestinal disease. J Pediatr 1981; 99:360–4.
63. Joly F, Dray X, Corcos O, et al. Tube feeding improves intestinal absorption in short bowel syndrome patients. Gastroenterology 2009;136:824–31.
64. Olieman JF, Penning C, Ijsselstijn H, et al. Enteral nutrition in children with short-bowel syndrome: current evidence and recommendations for the clinician. J Am Diet Assoc 2010;110:420–6.
65. Weber TR. Enteral feeding increases sepsis in infants with short bowel syndrome. J Pediatr Surg 1995;30(7):1086–8 [discussion: 1088–9].
66. Aynsley-Green A, Adrian TE, Bloom SR. Feeding and the development of enteroinsular hormone secretion in the preterm infant: effects of continuous gastric infusions of human milk compared with intermittent boluses. Acta Paediatr Scand 1982;71(3):379–83.
67. Braegger C, Decsi T, Dias JA, et al. Practical approach to paediatric enteral nutrition: a comment by the ESPGHAN committee on nutrition. J Pediatr Gastroenterol Nutr 2010;51:110–22.
68. Dahms BB, Halpin TC Jr. Serial liver biopsies in parenteral nutrition-associated cholestasis of early infancy. Gastroenterology 1981;81:136–44.
69. Lauriti G, Zani A, Aufieri R, et al. Incidence, prevention, and treatment of parenteral nutrition-associated cholestasis and intestinal failure-associated liver disease in infants and children: a systematic review. JPEN J Parenter Enteral Nutr 2014;38:70–85.
70. Farmer DG, Venick RS. Morbidity and mortality associated with chronic intestinal failure. Transplantation 2008;85(10):1385–6.
71. D'Antiga L, Goulet O. Intestinal failure in children: the European view. J Pediatr Gastroenterol Nutr 2013;56(2):118–26.
72. Lee WS, Sokol RJ. Intestinal microbiota, lipids, and the pathogonesis of intestinal failure-associated liver disease. J Pediatr 2015;167(3):519–26.
73. Diamond IR, de Silva NT, Tomlinson GA, et al. The role of parenteral lipids in the development of advanced intestinal failure-associated liver disease in infants: a multiple-variable analysis. JPEN J Parenter Enteral Nutr 2011;35:596–602.
74. Cober MP, Killu G, Brattain A. Intravenous fat emulsions reduction for patients with parenteral nutrition-associated liver disease. J Pediatr 2012;160(3):421–7.
75. Gura KM, Duggan CP, Collier SB, et al. Reversal of parenteral nutrition-associated liver disease in two infants with short bowel syndrome using parenteral fish oil: implications for future management. Pediatrics 2006;118(1):e197–201.

76. Premkumar MH, Carter BA, Hawthorne KM, et al. High rates of resolution of cholestasis in parenteral nutrition-associated liver disease with fish oil-based lipid emulsion monotherapy. J Pediatr 2013;162(4):793–8.
77. Calkins KL, Dunn JCY, Shew SB, et al. Pediatric intestinal failure–associated liver disease is reversed with 6 months of intravenous fish oil. JPEN J Parenter Enteral Nutr 2013;2013:1–11.
78. Belza C, Fitzgerald K, de Silva N, et al. Predicting intestinal adaptation in pediatric intestinal failure: a Retrospective Cohort Study. Ann Surg 2017. https://doi.org/10.1097/SLA.0000000000002602.
79. Colomb V, Fabeiro M, Dabbas M, et al. Central venous catheter-related infections in children on long-term home parenteral nutrition: incidence and risk factors. Clin Nutr 2000;19:355–9.
80. Buchman AL, Moukarzel A, Goodson B, et al. Catheter-related infections associated with home parenteral nutrition and predictive factors for the need for catheter removal in their treatment. JPEN J Parenter Enteral Nutr 1994;18:297–302.
81. Wales PW, Aleen N, Worthington P, et al. Clinical guidelines: support of pediatric patients with intestinal failure at risk of parenteral nutrition-associated liver disease. JPEN J Parenter Enteral Nutr 2014;38:538–57.
82. Chu HP, Brind J, Tomar R, et al. Significant reduction in central venous catheter-related bloodstream infections in children on HPN after starting treatment with taurolidine line lock. J Pediatr Gastroenterol Nutr 2012;55:403–7.
83. Cober MP, Kovacevich DS, Teitelbaum DH. Ethanol-lock therapy for the prevention of central venous access device infections in pediatric patients with intestinal failure. JPEN J Parenter Enteral Nutr 2011;35(1):67–73.
84. Cole CR, Frem JC, Schmotzer B, et al. The rate of bloodstream infection is high in infants with short bowel syndrome: relationship with small bowel bacterial overgrowth, enteral feeding, and inflammatory and immune responses. J Pediatr 2010;156(6):941–7.
85. Grant D, Abu-Elmagd K, Mazariegos G, et al, Intestinal Transplant Association. Intestinal transplant registry report: global activity and trends. Am J Transplant 2015;15(1):210–9.
86. Merritt R, Cohran V, Raphael B, et al. Intestinal rehabilitation programs in the management of pediatric intestinal failure and short bowel syndrome. J Pediatr Gastroenterol Nutr 2017;65:588–96.
87. Avitzur Y, Wang JY, de Silva NT, et al. Impact of intestinal rehabilitation program and its innovative therapies on the outcome of intestinal transplant candidates. J Pediatr Gastroenterol Nutr 2015;61(1):18–23.
88. Stanger JD, Oliveira C, Blackmore C, et al. The impact of multi-disciplinary intestinal rehabilitation programs on the outcome of pediatric patients with intestinal failure: a systematic review and meta-analysis. J Pediatr Surg 2013;48(5):983–92.
89. Fitzgibbons S, Ching YA, Valim C, et al. Relationship between serum citrulline levels and progression to parenteral nutrition independence in children with short bowel syndrome. J Pediatr Surg 2009;44:928–32.
90. Rhoads JM, Plunkett E, Galanko J, et al. Serum citrulline levels correlate with enteral tolerance and bowel length in infants with short bowel syndrome. J Pediatr 2005;146:542–7.
91. Jeppesen PB. Clinical significance of GLP-2 in short-bowel syndrome. J Nutr 2003;133:3721–4.
92. Jeppesen PB, Sanguinetti EL, Buchman A, et al. Teduglutide (ALX-0600), a dipeptidyl peptidase IV resistant glucagon-like peptide 2 analogue, improves intestinal function in short bowel syndrome patients. Gut 2005;54:1224–31.

93. O'Keefe SJ, Jeppesen PB, Gilroy R, et al. Safety and efficacy of teduglutide after 52 weeks of treatment in patients with short bowel intestinal failure. Clin Gastroenterol Hepatol 2013;11:815–23.e1-3.

94. Jeppesen PB, Gilroy R, Pertkiewicz M, et al. Randomised placebo-controlled trial of teduglutide in reducing parenteral nutrition and/or intravenous fluid requirements in patients with short bowel syndrome. Gut 2011;60:902–14.

95. Carter BA, Cohran VC, Cole CR, et al. Outcomes from a 12-week, open-label, multicenter clinical trial of teduglutide in pediatric short bowel syndrome. J Pediatr 2017;181:102–11.e5.

Management of the Patient with Chronic Intestinal Pseudo-Obstruction and Intestinal Failure

Loris Pironi, MD*, Anna Simona Sasdelli, MD

KEYWORDS

- Chronic intestinal pseudo-obstruction • Chronic intestinal failure
- Home parenteral nutrition • Enteral nutrition • Prokinetic agents • Stoma

KEY POINTS

- Chronic intestinal pseudo-obstruction (CIPO) is a severe form of intestinal dysmotility disorder, characterized by the impairment of gastrointestinal propulsion of the gut content in the absence of occluding lesions.
- CIPO is classified as primary, when no demonstrable etiopathogenetic cause is detected, and secondary to a variety of diseases.
- The diagnostic workup aims to identify the causes, to understand the pathophysiologic features and to address the therapy.
- Treatment is challenging, based on nutritional, pharmacologic, and surgical therapy and requires a multidisciplinary approach.
- A chronic intestinal failure requiring long-term home parenteral nutrition as primary life-saving therapy develops in 20% to 50% of patients with CIPO.

DEFINITION OF CHRONIC INTESTINAL PSEUDO-OBSTRUCTION AND CHRONIC INTESTINAL FAILURE

Chronic intestinal pseudo-obstruction (CIPO) represents the most severe form of intestinal dysmotility disorders, a term used to indicate a group of diseases characterized by the "presence of impaired gastrointestinal propulsion of the gut content in the absence of fixed occluding lesions."[1–4] The diagnosis of CIPO relies on the finding of chronic/recurrent obstructive type symptoms with radiological features of dilated intestine with air/fluid levels in the absence of any lumen-occluding lesion.[1–3] The

Disclosure: None.

Chronic Intestinal Failure Unit, Department of Medical and Surgical Sciences, Saint Orsola Hospital, University of Bologna, Bologna, Italy

* Corresponding author.

E-mail address: loris.pironi@unibo.it

main clinical features are recurrent/chronic episodes of intestinal occlusion with abdominal pain, nausea, and vomiting. Intestinal malrotation and small and large bowel volvulus are frequent onset events in children. Constant abdominal viscerosomatic pain is present in almost all the adults and in one-third of children, as allodynia (painful sensation evoked by physiologic levels of provocation) and hyperalgesia (more painful symptoms for the same level of painful stimulus). An involvement of the urinary tract may be present, more frequently in children, with bladder adynamia, megacystis and ureterohydronephrosis (megacystis-microcolon–intestinal hypoperistalsis syndrome).[4,5] In the last decades, the term "enteric dysmotility" (ED) has been proposed to describe patients with objective evidence of altered small bowel motility but without radiological features of a dilated intestine.[2,6] The outcome of ED and CIPO has been reported to differ greatly, with a higher risk to develop chronic intestinal failure (CIF) in CIPO, due to intolerance to oral or enteral nutrition, resulting in inadequate nutritional intake.[7,8] CIF is the type III intestinal failure, defined as the "persistent reduction of gut function below the minimum necessary for the absorption of macronutrients and/or water and electrolytes, such that intravenous supplementation is required to maintain health and/or growth."[3] Long-term home parenteral nutrition (HPN) is the life-saving therapy for CIF.[9,10] The term "intestinal insufficiency" (or "deficiency") has been proposed to classify patients with a reduction of gut function impairing intestinal absorption but in whom health and growth can be maintained by diet counseling, enteral tube feeding (ETF), vitamins, and trace element administration.[3]

EPIDEMIOLOGY AND CLASSIFICATION OF CHRONIC INTESTINAL PSEUDO-OBSTRUCTION

CIPO is a rare disease that can develop in both children and adults. Differences and similarities between adult and pediatric intestinal pseudo-obstruction have been recently highlighted.[5] Various CIPO classifications are reported in the literature.[2–4] CIPO is considered primary/idiopathic, when no underlying disorder can be demonstrated, or secondary, when related to a variety of systemic diseases, such as infections, autoimmune processes, mitochondrial dysfunction, either sporadic or familial, as well as side effects of medications[2–4] (Table 1). Secondary CIPO is rare in children and accounts for up to 50% in adults.[5] Primary CIPO develops in the neonatal age in about one-half of pediatric cases and appears mostly between 20 to 40 years of age in adults.[2,4–6] Epidemiologic studies in Japan reported a prevalence of 0.8 and 1.0 and an incidence of 0.21 and 0.24 cases per 100,000 adult men and women, respectively[11] and a prevalence of 3.7 per million children younger than 15 years.[12] CIPO accounts for around 20% of both adults and children on long-term HPN for CIF.[10,13,14] CIPO can be subdivided histologically into neuropathy (involving the enteric nervous system and/or the autonomic nervous system), myopathies (involving the smooth muscle), or mesenchymopathies (involving the interstitial cells of Cajal), with neuropathy representing the most frequent form.[2–4,15,16]

DIAGNOSIS OF CHRONIC INTESTINAL PSEUDO-OBSTRUCTION

The diagnosis of CIPO is primarily based on clinical and plain abdominal radiography feature. Imaging (entero-computed tomography and entero-magnetic resonance), gastrointestinal transit and manometry studies, endoscopic evaluations, generic and disease-specific laboratory tests, metabolic screening, neurologic evaluation, genetic tests and histopathology analysis on full-thickness intestinal biopsies are required to differentiate primary and secondary CIPO as well as myopathic and neuropathic CIPO, to know the gastrointestinal (GI) tracts affected by motility impairment and to

Table 1
Classification of chronic intestinal pseudo-obstruction

Onset Classification	Histopathologic Classification	Etiopathogenetic Classification
Congenital (present at birth) • Sporadic • Familial Acquired Pediatric • Neonatal onset: from prenatal to 12 mo of age • Late onset: from 1 to 18 y of age (sporadic cases) Adult • Median age of onset: 20–40 y	• Neuropathy: injury of the enteric nervous system • Myopathy: injury of the smooth muscle • Mesenchymopathy: injury of the interstitial cells of Cajal Inflammatory (mainly lymphocytic) neuro-muscular infiltrate may be present in all the categories	Primary/idiopathic: no demonstrable etiopathogenetic causes Secondary: with demonstrable etiopathogenetic causes • Autoimmune (ie, antibodies against membrane receptors; antibodies against gangliosides) • Collagen vascular diseases (ie, primary systemic sclerosis-scleroderma, systemic lupus erythematosus, dermatomyositis/polymyositis, periarteritis nodosa, rheumatoid arthritis, mixed connective tissue disorders, Ehlers-Danlos syndrome) • Endocrine disorders (ie: hypothyroidism, hypoparathyroidism, hyperparathyroidism) • Diabetes • Neurologic disorders (ie: Parkinson disease, Alzheimer disease, Shy-Drager syndrome, Chagas disease, Hirschsprung disease, dysautonomia, Von Recklinghausen disease, multiple sclerosis, myasthenia gravis, syringomyelia, and Guillain-Barrè syndrome) • Muscular dystrophies (ie: myotonic dystrophy, Duchenne muscular dystrophy) • Paraneoplastic (ie: central nervous system neoplasms, lung microcytoma, bronchial carcinoid, leiomyosarcomas, carcinoid, thymoma) • Amyloidosis • Infections (ie: Herpes Zoster virus, polyomaviruses, rotavirus, cytomegalovirus, Epstein–Barr virus, or other neurotropic viruses; Chagas disease, Lyme disease) • Mitochondrial disorders (ie: mitochondrial neurogastrointestinal encephalomyopathy (MNGIE); mitochondrial encephalomyopathy, lactic acidosis, and stroke (MELAS); Alper disease; POLG–DNA polymerase-gamma mutation) • Iatrogenic (ie: opioids, tricyclic antidepressants, anticholinergic agents, ganglionic blockers, anti-Parkinsonian agents, clonidine, phenothiazines) • Miscellaneous (ie: celiac disease, radiation enteritis, inflammatory bowel disease, chronic intestinal vascular insufficiency, eosinophilic gastroenteritis, fetal alcohol syndrome)

Data from Refs.[2–5]

identify cases of fabricated/induced illness by careers (Munchausen by proxy syndrome) in children.[2,4,5,15] The diagnostic investigations for CIPO are described in **Table 2**.

OUTCOME OF CHRONIC INTESTINAL PSEUDO-OBSTRUCTION

Studies on the outcome of CIPO show a higher mortality in children than in adults and in secondary than in primary CIPO.[5,16] In primary CIPO, onset at birth, acute onset of the disease, myogenic cause, occurrence of intestinal malrotation, presence of urinary tract involvement, and repeated surgery were observed risk factors for a poor prognosis.[16] The percentage of patients requiring HPN for CIF has been reported to range from 20% to 50% in adults and greater than 80% in children, in whom it is more frequent in the neonatal onset form.[5,6,17–19] The reversibility of CIF with weaning from HPN has been observed in 25% to 50% of adults and 25% to 38% in children,[5,16,18–20] whereas the mean 5-year survival probability on HPN was 70% (range: 48%–90%) in adults and 76% (65%–87%) in children, with a poorer outcome in secondary CIPO (systemic sclerosis: 5-year survival 18%).[5,16,19,20]

MANAGEMENT

Management of CIPO aims to improve the gut function, relieve the gastrointestinal symptoms, and maintain adequate nutritional status. The improvement of patient's quality of life (QoL) and the maintaining/development of the patient school life, education, and working career as well as social relationships and family life environment are the expected consequences of a successful treatment. Management of CIPO is based on nutrition and pharmacologic and surgical intervention. A multidisciplinary team, primarily including gastroenterologist, nutritionist, and surgeons who cooperate with the other medical specialists (psychologist, urologist, geneticist/metabolic medicine, general practitioner/pediatrician) and health care professionals (nurses, social workers, pharmacists) according to specific requirements of the single patient, is mandatory to optimize the result of treatment.[2,4,5,9]

PHARMACOLOGIC AND SURGICAL THERAPY

Pharmacologic therapy aims to improve GI motility, suppress bacterial overgrowth, and control intestinal inflammation and abdominal pain. The beneficial effects of drug treatment must be tested in individual patients. This indicates that pharmacologic trial should always be attempted, but there are no general rules and no expected outcome can be predicted.[1,2,4,5] Trials to improve GI motility with prokinetic agents are recommended in any patient (**Table 3**).[2–5,9]

Small intestinal bacterial overgrowth (SIBO) is a frequent complication in these patients.[8] SIBO causes mucosal inflammation, which further impairs GI motility. The European Society for Clinical Nutrition and Metabolism (ESPEN) guidelines for CIF in adults suggest periodic and rotating cycles of antibiotic therapy to prevent SIBO in patients with CIPO who have frequent relapsing episodes. The antibiotic choice for SIBO is empiric. Nonabsorbable antibiotics should be the first choice, such as rifaximin or aminoglycosides by oral route, but broad-spectrum antibiotics (amoxicillin and clavulanic acid, metronidazole, fluoroquinolones, doxycycline, sometimes associated with an antifungal compound) are also used.[5,9]

Patients may require drugs to relieve visceral pain. Low doses of antidepressants (tricyclic antidepressants or the noradrenergic serotonergic reuptake inhibitors) and/or gabapentinoids (gabapentin and pregabalin) are prescribed.[4] Opioids should be

Table 2
The diagnostic investigations for chronic idiopathic pseudo-obstruction

Diagnostic Test	Aims and Comments
Plain abdominal radiography	First screening to identify dilated intestinal loops and air-fluid levels
Imaging studies • Small bowel follow-through with water-soluble contrast (SBPT) • Entero-computed tomography (ECT) • Entero-MRI (E-MRI)	To exclude malrotation and organic lesions occluding the gut SBPT: contrast material flocculation in the dilated intestinal loops ECT and E-MRI to be preferred
Urinary tract imaging	To evaluate urinary tract involvement
Gastric empting assessment • Food labeled scintigraphy • C13 breath test • Wireless motility capsule test • Cine-MRI Measurement of gut transit time (radio-opaque markers)	To detect/exclude gastroparesis To differentiate between functional constipation and nonretentive fecal incontinence
Manometry Antroduodenal manometry Colonic manometry Oesophageal manometry Anorectal manometry	To differentiate a pseudo-obstructive syndrome from a mechanical obstruction To differentiate enteric neuropathy from enteric myopathy To predict/assess the clinical response to pharmacologic treatment and the tolerance to enteral tube feeding To assess the extent of the disease To evaluate whether a defunctioning ileostomy might increase oral/enteral tube feeding tolerability Before intestinal transplantation, to evaluate whether the colon should be conserved To assess the extent of the disease To rule out Hirschsprung disease Before intestinal transplantation, to evaluate whether the colon should be conserved
Radio-opaque marker study	To assess intestinal transit time
Breath testing H_2 breath test (Lactose) or $13CO_2$ breath test	To detect small intestinal bacterial overgrowth (to be interpreted in light of small bowel transit)
Endoscopy	To exclude a mechanical occlusion To identify secondary diseases
Surgical exploration	To confirm or exclude the presence of a mechanical occlusion of the gut
Histopathology	Bowel full-thickness or near full-thickness biopsy is required to examine nerve, muscle, and interstitial cells of Cajal. Specimens taken during emergency or planned surgical resection or ad hoc laparoscopic surgery Differentiation between myopathic and neuropathic is useful for the prognosis
Laboratory tests and metabolic screening	To evaluate secondary forms of CIPO

(continued on next page)

Table 2 (continued)	
Diagnostic Test	**Aims and Comments**
Genetic tests	Search for:
	CAID syndrome (SGOL 1 mutation)
	ACTG2 gene–associated megacystis–microcolon–intestinal hypoperistalsis syndrome.
	MNGIE
	MELAS
	Alper disease, POLG–DNA polymerase-gamma mutation
	Others
Neurologic evaluation	To evaluate secondary forms of CIPO
Autonomic function testing	To differentiate between gastrointestinal and generalized autonomic disturbance, in patients with signs or symptoms of dysautonomia

Data from Refs.[2–5]

used only and carefully in nonresponsive patients with untreatable pain, because they may further impair the GI motility. Tramadol and codeine have no effect on gastroenteric and small bowel motility, but at equianalgesic doses, tramadol causes less delay in colon transit than codeine.[4] Steroids and immunosuppressive drugs (eg, azathioprine) might be an effective therapeutic option in cases of histopathologic signs of marked inflammation.[4,5]

Nontransplant surgery may be required for explorative laparotomy to exclude mechanical obstruction; for intestinal resection; and for creating a venting/feeding gastrostomy, a jejunostomy, and a decompressive ileostomy or colostomy. Decompressive procedures reduce the degree of abdominal distension and may alleviate obstructive symptoms and increase the tolerance of enteral feeding. Early small intestine decompression in the course of the disease is advisable, because it allows to preserve as much as possible the already compromised motor function of the gut and limits further deterioration. On the contrary, it is recommended to avoid unnecessary surgeries, because of the high risk of dense adhesions after surgery and prolonged postsurgical paralytic ileus observed in these patients.[1,2,4,5]

NUTRITIONAL THERAPY

Nutrition therapy plays a primary role in CIPO because gastrointestinal motility is further impaired by the presence of malnutrition, dehydration, and electrolyte deficiency (namely sodium, potassium, and magnesium), whereas optimal nutritional status allows to maximize the residual gut function.[5] Oral feeding, ETF (bolus or continuous), and HPN should be tailored to each patient. Dietary counseling should be the first-line management[9,21] and may be sufficient for patients with mild and moderate dysmotility. The oral intake of patients with CIPO is influenced by the extent of gastrointestinal disease. It may be more limited in patients with gastroparesis who often complain of early satiety, bloating, and nausea, than in patients with predominantly small bowel involvement.[22] The oral diet should aim to optimize gut motility by minimizing the postprandial digestive workload and to decrease the risk of SIBO and gastric bezoar. This may require low-fiber, low-fat, low-lactose, and

Table 3
Prokinetic agents for the treatment of chronic intestinal pseudo-obstruction

Drug	Mechanism	Dosage	Comment
Amoxicillin/ Clavulanate	Increased small bowel contractions via propogation of phase III migrating motor complexes	P: 20 mg/kg up to antibiotic dose A: 500–1000 mg 3 times daily, 30 min before meals	Mechanism of action still not well defined
Erythromycin	Motilin receptor agonist	P: 3–5 mg/kg A: 50–500 mg orally or 50–100 mg intravenously (iv) 3–4 times daily, 30 min before meals	Contraindicated with cytochrome P4503A4 inhibitors
Azithromycin	Motilin receptor agonist	P: 10 mg/kg A: 500 mg Once daily	Longer duration of effect than erythromycin Azithromycin does not have significant drug–drug interactions
Metoclopramide	Dopamine-2 (D2) receptor antagonist at chemoreceptor trigger zone 5HT4 agonist in the gut	P: 0.4–0.8 mg/kg (up to 10 mg) per dose A: 10 mg per dose 3–4 times daily	Cause hyperprolactinemia Able to cross blood-brain barrier with extrapyramidal reaction
Cisapride	5HT4 agonist with acetylcholine release in the gut	P: 0.2–0.3 mg/kg max 10 mg) A: 10 mg 3–4 times daily 30 min before meals	Cisapride has been withdrawn due to risk of cardiac arrhythmias due to QTc interval prolongation
Domperidone	Dopamine-2 (D2) receptor antagonist in the gut	P 0.1–0.3 mg/kg, max dose 10–20 mg A: 10–20 mg 2–4 times daily, 30 min before meals	Causes QTc interval prolongation and hyperprolactinemia Unable to cross blood-brain barrier
Bethanechol	Cholinergic acting on muscarinic receptor	P: 0.1–0.2 mg/kg A: 10–50 mg 4 times daily	
Neostigmine	Acetylcholinesterase inhibitor	P: 0.01–0.05 mg/kg per dose (iv repeated at suitable intervals, max 5) A: 1 mg single dose	
Pyridostigmine	Acetylcholinesterase inhibitor	P: start with 0.1–0.3 mg/kg per dose 2–3 times daily and increase as tolerated	

(continued on next page)

Table 3 (continued)			
Drug	**Mechanism**	**Dosage**	**Comment**
		A: max 30 mg b.i.d. orally	
Octreotide	Somatostatin analogue Induces migrating motor complex propagation in the small bowel	P: 0.5–1 μg/kg A: 25–50 μg Subcutaneously after both the morning and evening meals	Useful in CIPO due to scleroderma and in paraneoplastic CIPO Improves small bowel motility, but decreases gastric motility
Prucalopride	5-hydroxytryptamine receptor 4 (5HT4)	P: 0.02–0.04 mg/kg per d up to 2 mg/d A: 2–4 mg/d	

Abbreviations: A, adult; P, pediatric.
   Data from Refs.[2–5]

low-fructose diet composed of soft foods and divided into 5 to 6 small frequent meals.[5,9] In order to meet an adequate caloric intake, oral supplement formulae can be helpful, if tolerated.[5,9,21,22] Patients with CIPO may also be at risk of developing vitamin and trace element deficiencies (ie, iron, zinc, folate, vitamin D, and vitamin B12); therefore, multivitamin preparations should be added to their diet. In patients with severe gastrointestinal dysmotility, supplemental or total ETF may be required to meet their nutritional needs and to avoid weight loss. A few day trial of nasogastric or nasojejunal ETF is required to assess if the patient is able to tolerate the formula and the rate of formula delivery (bolus or continuous). Then, temporary or permanent percutaneous endoscopic gastrostomy (with or without jejunal extension) or a jejunostomy can be positioned by endoscopic, surgical, and radiological placement.[1,2] The modality of ETF and the type of formula need to be tailored to the patient's tolerance and requirements. The few reports on ETF in patients with CIPO are on children.[5,9] In gastric ETF, continuous and low rate infusion through a peristaltic pump, rather than bolus infusion, could be required to avoid abdominal bloating and nausea. In cases of severe gastroparesis, a venting gastrostomy can be added to the jejunostomy.[5,9] Jejunal ETF should always be performed by continuous infusion. The tolerance of jejunal ETF has been shown to be more likely in children with normal fasting enteric motility represented by the presence of phase 3 of the migrating motor complexes in duodenum or jejunum.[23] Polymeric and normal/low osmolality ETF formula should be used in both jejunal and gastric feeding. However, even though ETF should be attempted in patients with motility disorders, clinical experience suggests a low rate of long-term tolerance.[24]

LONG-TERM HOME PARENTERAL NUTRITION FOR CHRONIC INTESTINAL FAILURE

Drug therapy, surgical procedures, dietary counseling, and ETF are successful to maintain nutritional status in around two-thirds of patients with CIPO, who are therefore categorized as having "intestinal insufficiency/deficiency," whereas one-third develops CIF, requiring long-term HPN.[3,5,9,17–19] The ESPEN gives recommendations for the management of HPN for CIF as well as for the management of the underlying intestinal pathology and the prevention and treatment of the major HPN-related complications.[9] The outcome of primary CIPO with CIF has been described in terms of survival rate, causes of death, risk of major HPN complications, QoL, and probability of intestinal rehabilitation. The survival rate on HPN has increased in the recent decades, probably due to the better understanding and management of the disease as well as the management of HPN. A 5-year survival of greater than or equal to 80% has been consistently reported in both adults and children, a feature that is similar or even better than that of patients with CIF due to other diseases.[8,19,20,25] A review of the literature showed that in adults with CIPO, the causes of death on HPN did not differ from those observed in patients with CIF due to other underlying diseases, being related to HPN major complications in 6% of cases, the underlying disease in 57%, and to other causes in 36%.[16] Ability to restore oral feeding and age at disease onset less than 20 years were associated with a lower risk of death, whereas secondary CIPO showed an increased risk.[16] A greater percentage of HPN-related death was observed in the neonatal age[16] but not in older children.[19] Neonatal and acute onset of the disease, occurrence of intestinal malrotation, urinary involvement, and the myopathic origin of CIPO were factors associated with an increased risk of death.[16] A recent multicenter international study investigated QoL using a specific questionnaire for adult patients on HPN for CIF (HPN-QOL).[26] The results showed that patients with CIPO had a lower QoL than those having Crohn disease or mesenteric ischemia as underlying disease.[26] Studies in children have given contrasting results showing QoL either equal to or lower than that of healthy controls.[5] Up to date, no factors associated with a higher probability of CIF reversibility in CIPO have been clearly demonstrated.[5,8,20]

TRANSPLANTATION IN PATIENTS WITH CHRONIC INTESTINAL PSEUDO-OBSTRUCTION

Four types of transplantation have been performed in patients with CIPO: intestinal transplantation (ITx), allogeneic hematopoietic stem cell transplantation (AHSCT), orthotopic liver transplantation (OLT), and fecal microbiota transplantation (FMT). The ESPEN guidelines recommend that only patients with impending or overt liver failure due to intestinal failure associated liver disease and those with an invasive intra-abdominal desmoid tumor be listed for a "life-saving" ITx.[9] Also patients with central venous catheter–related thrombosis occluding of 2 or more central veins might be considered candidates for a life-saving ITx, but only on a careful case-by-case basis.[9] Indeed, outcome data clearly demonstrated that patients with CIF due to CIPO have a rate of survival on HPN that favorably compare with post-ITx survival, that is reported to range from 50% to 70% at 5 year, mostly depending on the ITx center expertise.[9,16,27–29] Therefore, patients with CIPO would be rarely listed for a life-saving ITx. The ESPEN guidelines suggest that a so-called "rehabilitative" ITx might be considered in patients with CIF with high morbidity or low acceptance of HPN on a careful case-by-case basis.[9]

AHSCT and OLT are the curative treatment options for mitochondrial neurogastrointestinal encephalomyopathy (MNGIE), an ultra-rare cause of secondary CIPO.[30,31] MNGIE is an autosomal recessive disease caused by mutations in the nuclear TYMP gene, leading to a marked reduction or absence of thymidine phosphorylase (TP) activity, resulting in a systemic toxic accumulation of nucleosides thymidine and deoxyuridine, which induces progressive mitochondrial DNA damage.[32] AHSCT and OLT are the life-saving TP replacement therapy for these patients otherwise destined to die.

Recently, a pilot study on 9 adult patients suggested that serial FMT may be a candidate therapy for CIPO.[33] FMT transfers stool from healthy donors to patients with an altered colonic microbiome with the aim to cure a specific disease.[34] FMT significantly alleviated abdominal symptoms, improved ETF toleration, reduced Computed To-mography scores of intestinal obstructions and eliminated SIBO almost all patients.[33] Further studies are required to confirm if this could be an effective therapy for patients with CIPO and to define criteria for optimal candidates to the treatment.

SUMMARY

CIPO is a severe form of intestinal dysmotility disorder, characterized by the impairment of gastrointestinal propulsion of the gut content in the absence of occluding lesions. The etiopathogenetic classification categorizes CIPO as primary, when no demonstrable cause is detected and secondary to a variety of disease. CIPO can be due to damage of the enteric nervous system (neuropathy), smooth muscle (myopathy), and/or interstitial cells of Cajal (mesenchymopathy). The diagnostic workup aims to identify the causes, understand the pathophysiologic features, and address the therapy. Treatment of CIPO is challenging and is based on nutritional, pharmacologic, and surgical therapy and requires a multidisciplinary approach. A CIF requiring long-term HPN as primary life-saving therapy develops in 20% to 50% of patients with CIPO. The patient survival rate is good, but the effectiveness of treatments in improving gastrointestinal function and relieving symptoms is often not satisfactory.

REFERENCES

1. Frances LC, Di Lorenzo C. Chronic intestinal pseudo-obstruction: assessment and management. Gastroenterology 2006;130:S29–36.
2. Paine P, McLaughlin J, Lal S. Review article: the assessment and management of chronic severe gastrointestinal dysmotility in adults. Aliment Pharmacol Ther 2013;38(10):1209–29.
3. Pironi L, Arends J, Baxter J, et al. Home Artificial Nutrition & Chronic Intestinal Failure; Acute Intestinal Failure Special Interest Groups of ESPEN. ESPEN endorsed recommendations. Definition and classification of intestinal failure in adults. Clin Nutr 2015;34(2):171–80.
4. Di Nardo G, Di Lorenzo C, Lauro A, et al. Chronic intestinal pseudo-obstruction in children and adults: diagnosis and therapeutic options. Neurogastroenterol Motil 2017;29(1). https://doi.org/10.1111/nmo.12945.
5. Thapar N, Saliakellis E, Benninga MA, et al. Paediatric Intestinal Pseudo-obstruction: Evidence and Consensus-based Recommendations From an ESPGHAN-Led Expert Group. J Pediatr Gastroenterol Nutr 2018;66(6):991–1019.
6. Wingate D, Hongo M, Kellow J, et al. Disorders of gastrointestinal motility: Towards a new classification. J Gastroenterol Hepatol 2002;17(s1):S1–4.
7. Lindberg G, Iwarzon M, Törnblom H. Clinical features and long-term survival in chronic intestinal pseudo-obstruction and enteric dysmotility. Scand J Gastroenterol 2009;44(6):692–9.
8. Vasant DH, Kalaiselvan R, Ablett J, et al. The chronic intestinal pseudo-obstruction subtype has prognostic significance in patients with severe gastrointestinal dysmotility related intestinal failure. Clin Nutr 2018;37(6 Pt A):1967–75.
9. Pironi L, Arends J, Bozzetti F, et al. ESPEN guidelines on chronic intestinal failure in adults. Clin Nutr 2016;35(2):247–307.
10. Pironi L, Konrad D, Brandt C, et al. Clinical classification of adult patients with chronic intestinal failure due to benign disease: an international multicenter cross-sectional survey. Clin Nutr 2018;37(2):728–38.

11. Lida H, Ohkudo H, Inamori M, et al. Epidemiology and clinical experience on chronic intestinal pseudo-obstruction in Japan: a nationwide epidemiologic survey. J Epidemiol 2013;23:288–94.

12. Muto M, Matsufuji H, Tomomasa T, et al. Pediatric chronic intestinal pseudo-obstruction is a rare, serious, and intractable disease: a report of a nationwide survey in Japan. J Pediatr Surg 2014;49:1799–803.

13. Pironi L, Hébuterne X, Van Gossum A, et al. Candidates for intestinal transplantation: a multicenter survey in Europe. Am J Gastroenterol 2006;101(7):1633–43 [quiz: 1679].

14. Diamanti A, Capriati T, Gandullia P, et al. Pediatric Chronic Intestinal Failure in Italy: Report from the 2016 Survey on Behalf of Italian Society for Gastroenterology, Hepatology and Nutrition (SIGENP). Nutrients 2017;9(11) [pii:E1217].

15. Knowles CH, De Giorgio R, Kapur RP, et al. The London Classification of gastrointestinal neuromuscular pathology: report on behalf of the Gastro 2009 International Working Group. Gut 2010;59:882–7.

16. Pironi L, Goulet O, Buchman A, et al. Home Artificial Nutrition and Chronic Intestinal Failure Working Group of ESPEN. Outcome on home parenteral nutrition for benign intestinal failure: a review of the literature and benchmarking with the European prospective survey of ESPEN [Review]. Clin Nutr 2012;31(6):831–45.

17. Stanghellini V, Cogliandro RF, De Giorgio R, et al. Natural history of chronic idiopathic intestinal pseudo-obstruction in adults: a single center study. Clin Gastroenterol Hepatol 2005;3:449–58.

18. Faure C, Goulet O, Ategbo S, et al. Chronic intestinal pseudoobstruction syndrome: clinical analysis, outcome, and prognosis in 105 children. French-Speaking Group of Pediatric Gastroenterology. Dig Dis Sci 1999;44:953–9.

19. Diamanti A, Fusaro F, Caldaro T, et al. Pediatric intestinal pseudo-obstruction: impact of neonatal and later onset on clinical and nutritional outcomes. J Pediatr Gastroenterol Nutr 2019. https://doi.org/10.1097/MPG.0000000000002373.

20. Amiot A, Joly F, Alves A, et al. Long-term outcome of chronic intestinal pseudo-obstruction adult patients requiring home parenteral nutrition. Am J Gastroenterol 2009;104:1262–70.

21. Billiauws L, Corcos O, Joly F. Dysmotility disorders: a nutritional approach. Curr Opin Clin Nutr Metab Care 2014;17(5):483–8.

22. Smith DS, Williams CS, Ferris CD. Diagnosis and treatment of chronic gastroparesis and chronic intestinal pseudo-obstruction. Gastroenterol Clin North Am 2003;32(2):619–58.

23. Di Lorenzo C, Flores AF, Buie T, et al. Intestinal motility and jejunal feeding in children with chronic intestinal pseudo-obstruction. Gastroenterology 1995;108: 1379–85.

24. Cucchiara S, Borrelli O. Nutritional challenge in pseudo-obstruction: the bridge between motility and nutrition. J Pediatr Gastroenterol Nutr 2000;48(Suppl. 2): S83–5.

25. Joly F, Baxter JI, Staun M, et al, ESPEN HAN CIF group. Five-year survival and causes of death in patients on home parenteral nutrition for severe chronic and benign intestinal failure. Clin Nutr 2018;37(4):1415–22.

26. Baxter JP, Fayers PM, Bozzetti F, et al. Home Artificial Nutrition and Chronic Intestinal Failure Special Interest Group of the European Society for Clinical Nutrition and Metabolism (ESPEN). An international study of the quality of life of adult patients treated with home parenteral nutrition. Clin Nutr 2018. https://doi.org/10.1016/j.clnu.2018.07.024.

27. Pironi L, Joly F, Forbes A, et al. Home Artificial Nutrition & Chronic Intestinal Failure Working Group of the European Society for Clinical Nutrition and Metabolism (ESPEN). Long-term follow-up of patients on home parenteral nutrition in Europe: implications for intestinal transplantation. Gut 2011;60(1):17–25.
28. Grant D, Abu-Elmagd K, Mazariegos G, et al. Intestinal transplant registry report: global activity and trends. Am J Transplant 2015;15(1):210–9.
29. Bharadwaj S, Tandon P, Gohel TD, et al. Current status of intestinal and multivisceral transplantation. Gastroenterol Rep (Oxf) 2017;5(1):20–8.
30. Hirano M, Marti R, Casali C, et al. Allogeneic stem cell transplantation corrects biochemical derangements in MNGIE. Neurology 2006;67:1458–60.
31. De Giorgio R, Pironi L, Rinaldi R, et al. Liver transplantation for mitochondrial neurogastrointestinal encephalomyopathy. Ann Neurol 2016;80(3):448–55.
32. Hirano M, Silvestri G, Blake DM, et al. Mitochondrial neurogastrointestinal encephalomyopathy (MNGIE): clinical, biochemical, and genetic features of an autosomal recessive mitochondrial disorder. Neurology 1994;44:721–7.
33. Gu L, Ding C, Tian H, et al. Serial frozen fecalmicrobiota transplantation in the treatment of chronic intestinal pseudo-obstruction: a preliminary study. J Neurogastroenterol Motil 2017;23:289–97.
34. Vindigni SM, Surawicz CM. Fecal microbiota transplantation. Gastroenterol Clin North Am 2017;46:171–85.

Weaning from Parenteral Nutrition

Andrew Ukleja, MD, AGAF

KEYWORDS

- Parenteral nutrition • Parenteral support • Short bowel syndrome • Intestinal failure
- Teduglutide (Gattex) • GLP-2 • Growth hormone • Treatment

KEY POINTS

- The ultimate goal in the treatment of short bowel syndrome-intestinal failure (SBS-IF) patients is to achieve enteral autonomy, thereby eliminating parenteral nutrition (PN) or intravenous fluids (IV).
- Weaning from PN/IV is a complex process that should be individualized for each patient, and attempt in a stable patient after the optimization process involving diet modification, oral hydration and conventional anti-diarrheal medications.
- Currently, teduglutide, GLP-2 analogue, is the preferred adjuvant agent for PN/IV weaning after unsuccessful attempts of weaning with standard approach.
- A majority of patients treated with teduglutide can expect significant reduction in PN/IV volumes, however, a limited number of patients can achieve full independence from PN/IV.
- Following PN/IV elimination, SBS-IF patients will need long-term monitoring for nutritional deficiencies.

INTRODUCTION

Intestinal failure (IF) is a consequence of extensive bowel resection, nonoperable obstruction, dysmotility, and congenital defects associated with insufficient functional gut capacity for adequate fluid and nutrient absorption, which results in a dependence on parenteral support (parenteral nutrition [PN] or intravenous [IV] fluids).[1,2] Short bowel syndrome (SBS) is the most common cause of IF, and many patients with SBS require long-term parenteral support. Although PN is a lifesaving therapy for patients with IF, it has been associated with serious life-threatening complications, such as catheter-related sepsis, vein thrombosis, and liver failure.[3,4] In a study by Amiot and colleagues,[5] 10-year survival was significantly worse among patients with SBS who remained dependent on PN in comparison with those who became independent from PN (10.7% vs

Disclosure Statement: Member of an advisory board for Coram, Therachon, and Shire (in the past).
Division of Gastroenterology and Hepatology, Beth Israel Deaconess Medical Center/Beth Israel Lahey Health, 330 Brookline Ave., Boston, MA 02215, USA
E-mail address: aukleja@bidmc.harvard.edu

Gastroenterol Clin N Am 48 (2019) 525–550
https://doi.org/10.1016/j.gtc.2019.08.007
0889-8553/19/© 2019 Elsevier Inc. All rights reserved.

67.0%; P = .001). In addition, reduced quality of life has been observed in PN-dependent patients, including disruptions in daily activities, sleep patterns, and social interactions.[6,7] Therefore, it is highly desirable to transition patients with SBS-IF from PN/IV to an oral diet. Achieving enteral autonomy should be the primary long-term goal for PN/IV-dependent patients with SBS. Traditionally, the best practice management strategies for patients with SBS-IF have been restricted to dietary interventions, optimization of hydration, and antidiarrheal pharmacotherapy (intestinal rehabilitation) to allow successful weaning from PN/IV. However, only a small percentage of patients treated with traditional management strategies were able to be weaned from PN/IV. In a study by Messing and colleagues,[8] 55% of adult patients with SBS on home parenteral support were weaned off within 5 years. Targeted pharmacotherapy was needed to augment intestinal adaptation and reduce the needs for PN/IV. Trophic agents, a growth hormone (GH), and teduglutide (glucagon-like peptide [GLP]-2 analogue) were found to be beneficial in promoting the PN/IV weaning process.[9–15] At present, teduglutide seems to be a preferred adjuvant agent for PN weaning in a clinical practice.

Weaning from PN/IV is a process of gradual reductions of PN/IV volume and/or calories, days off over variable time frame, during which the patient is able to maintain clinical stability, leading to complete PN/IV elimination. The gradual weaning strategy is recommended for most patients with SBS with PN dependency over an extended period of time, despite that some patients may successfully discontinue PN rapidly. Rapid PN discontinuation, over a few days, is not recommended because it may put patients at high risk of dehydration.

A paucity of publications addresses the PN weaning strategies for patients with SBS-IF. Those strategies are mainly based on expert opinions and general consensus instead of scientific evidence.[16–18] The process of PN weaning is complex and requires collaboration from the patient and the medical team. The approval of teduglutide for use in the clinical practice expanded PS weaning options for patients with SBS-IF. Treatment with teduglutide allowed for more patients to achieve enteral autonomy. The integration of teduglutide into weaning strategy also adds to the complexity of the PN/IV weaning process. It also calls for attention of health care providers to familiarize themselves with the current indications, limitations, and general concerns about the medication long-term effects. In clinical studies featuring teduglutide, well-designed protocol has been used allowing for the safe and gradual PN/IV volume reduction in patients with SBS-IF.[12,13] This protocol is applied to the weaning processes with or without teduglutide in the clinical practice. This article addresses the current approach to PN/IV weaning. The preweaning, during, and postweaning considerations allowing successful weaning from parenteral support are described.

GENERAL CONSIDERATIONS BEFORE PARENTERAL NUTRITION WEANING

The mismatch between the degree of intestinal adaptation and gut functional capacity after massive bowel resection, resulting in severe losses of nutrients and fluids, has a major impact on the degree of PN/IV requirements. Intestinal adaptation, desired natural compensatory process characterized by structural and functional changes in the intestine, leads to improved nutrient and fluid absorption in the remnant bowel over time.[19] This process is critical for the facilitation of PN/IV weaning, but it is enhanced further by using intestinotrophic agents, such as teduglutide (GLP-2 analogue) or GH. Traditionally, the success of PN/IV weaning is influenced by several factors, such as the health and length of the remnant bowel, the presence of a colon and/or ileocecal valve, the degree of bowel adaptation, patient's compliance with the diet, oral rehydration solutions (ORS), and pharmacotherapy. The predictors for the success of PN/IV weaning are shown in **Box 1**.[5,17] Although bowel anatomy, underlying disease, and the severity of SBS have a major impact on PN/IV weaning rate, other important factors must be considered before attempting weaning.

PATIENT-CLINICIAN COLLABORATION

Patient engagement in the PN weaning process is crucial. Successful PN weaning requires that the patient is properly educated about the process and motivated to succeed. The patient should have a good understanding of pathophysiologic changes associated with extensive bowel resection, and therapy goals and expectations. PN weaning requires the patient to be highly compliant with dietary interventions, oral rehydration, and his or her antidiarrheal regimen. These interventions are needed to maximize nutrient and fluid absorption in the remnant intestine and to prevent dehydration. PN/IV weaning strategy should be reviewed with the patient. It is helpful for the patients to keep a food diary to monitor their diet. With proper education, patients should be able to identify signs and symptoms of dehydration. Risks of weaning from PN are shown in **Box 2**. The monitoring of urine and stoma output and body weight should be initiated even before the start of the weaning process to assess patient compliance. Patients who are given consideration for teduglutide should have understanding of the goals and expectations of therapy, potential adverse effects, appropriate monitoring, and recommended testing to ensure a safe weaning process. In addition, patients should be aware of a need for close monitoring (blood work, office visits, telephone contacts) to confirm their compliance with the weaning protocol.

OPTIMIZATION PROCESS

The optimization process involves fluid and nutrient stabilization before any attempt at the weaning from PN. The patient's diet, oral hydration, and medications should be optimized to avoid dehydration and weight loss before starting the weaning process. The optimization of oral and/or enteral nutrition (EN) and oral hydration significantly increases the chance of successful PN/IV weaning.

Box 1
Factors associated with the success of parenteral support (PN/IV) weaning in short bowel syndrome/intestinal failure

- Length of the remnant functional small bowel: >75 cm
- Presence of a colon
- Presence of an ileocecal valve
- Absence of disease in the remnant bowel
- Degree of intestinal adaptation
- Higher fasting plasma citrulline levels: >20 mmol/dL
- Younger age of the patient
- Duration of parenteral support: <2 years
- Nutritional status before weaning attempt
- Patient compliant with diet, hydration, and antidiarrheal therapy

Data from Refs.[5–8]

Box 2
Risks of weaning from parenteral support

- Dehydration
- Renal insufficiency
- Electrolytes abnormalities (sodium, potassium, bicarbonates)
- Vitamin and mineral deficiencies (vitamin B_{12}, fat-soluble vitamins [A, D, E], magnesium, phosphorus, zinc)
- Essential fatty acids deficiency
- Weight loss
- Feeling tired/fatigue
- Kidney stones
- Hypotension

Diet Modifications

Oral nutrition plays a critical role in maximizing intestinal rehabilitation.[20] Diet has a major impact on the augmentation of nutrient and fluid absorption. In addition, it greatly influences the degree of diarrhea/stoma output. Complex luminal nutrients in food stimulate intestinal adaptation by enhancing the release of the trophic factor, promoting villi growth, improving blood flow to the gut, and stimulating pancreaticobiliary secretions.[19] The diet should be customized based on remnant bowel anatomy and an underlying disease (**Table 1**).

Table 1
Diet recommendations for patients with SBS-IF with and without colon

Diet Components	End-Jejunostomy or Ileostomy	Presence of Colon in Continuity
Carbohydrates	40%–50% complex carbohydrates Avoid simple sugars Modified FODMAP diet	50% complex carbohydrates Avoid simple sugars Modified FODMAP diet
Fat	30%–40% of energy Fat with high content of EFA preferred Limit MCT	>30% of energy Fat with high content of EFA preferred Consider MCT
Protein	20%–30%	20%–30%
Fiber	Standard dose	Soluble fiber 5–10 g/d is preferred
Fluids	ORS/high-sodium fluids Fluid restriction may be needed if high stoma output	ORS may be beneficial
Salt	Increase salt intake High-sodium food	Standard amount intake
Oxalate	No restriction	Limit Calcium supplementation (to bind oxalate as preventive measure)

Abbreviations: EFA, essential fatty acids; FODMAP, Fermentable Oligo-, Di-, Mono-saccharides and Polyols diet; MCT, medium-chain triglycerides.

Data from Byrne TA, Veglia LM, Camelio M, et al. Beyond the prescription: optimizing the diet of patients with short bowel syndrome. Nutr Clin Pract 2000;15:306-311 and Jeppesen PB, Fuglsang KA. Nutritional Therapy in Adult Short Bowel Syndrome Patients with Chronic Intestinal Failure. Gastroenterol Clin North Am 2018;47:61-75.

Patients with SBS with end stomas, without a colon, should follow a high-fat diet (30%–40% of calories).[21] In those patients, medium-chain triglyceride supplementation should be avoided because of that strategy's negative effects on protein and carbohydrate absorption in the gut.[22] More complex dietary modifications are required in patients with a colon in continuity.[23,24] A high complex carbohydrate diet (30%–40% of calories) is preferred. Soluble fiber (pectin) has especially beneficial effect by increasing colonic transit, bulking the stool, and serving as a substrate for bacterial fermentation in the colon.[25] Patients with a colon may be able to salvage up to 1000 calories daily from short-chain fatty acids produced from unabsorbed carbohydrates by bacterial fermentation.[26] In addition, a low-fat diet is recommended for patients with a colon in continuity to avoid steatorrhea. Patients with a colon should also restrict oxalates in their diets because of an increased risk of oxalate stone formation in the kidneys from the excessive colonic absorption of oxalates.[27] The combination of distal ileal resection (>100 cm), colon-in-continuity, and fat malabsorption results in an increased absorption of dietary oxalate in the colon. Decreased bile acid secretion as a result of a reduced bile acid pool from interruption in the enterohepatic circulation of bile acids causes malabsorption of fatty acids, which bind to calcium rather than oxalate, leaving free oxalate. High concentration of oxalate in the colon stimulates its absorption and leads to hyperoxaluria and renal stone formation.[28] Protein intake should be at 20% of the daily energy intake in all patients. In general, oral caloric intake should be high with recommended increase of up to 50% to correct fecal nutrient and energy losses. Hyperphagia should be encouraged to meet energy targets.[29] However, many patients with a colon in continuity may avoid higher oral intake because of a high risk of exacerbation of postprandial diarrhea as a result of the increased oral intake. In this situation, higher dosages of antidiarrheal medications should be considered to reduce diarrhea.

Oral Fluids/Oral Hydration

Maintaining hydration and preventing dehydration are important priorities for patients with SBS before and during the PS weaning process. Patients with proximal stomas (jejunostomy) are especially at high risk for dehydration. To counteract dehydration, patients should maintain sufficient fluid intake, at least 30 mL/kg/d.[16] Oral fluid intake for patients with end-jejunostomy or ileostomy should be greater than 2 L/d to meet or exceed stoma outputs. ORS have been used successfully to improve fluid absorption and to reduce the severity of diarrhea. These beneficial effects are the result of optimal sodium and glucose concentrations in oral fluids, allowing for the maximization of fluid absorption by using the sodium-glucose cotransport system in the gut.[30] ORS seem to be more advantageous for patients with end-stomas and those patients with severe fluid losses in whom a minor increase in oral intake may have a major impact on stoma/stool output. Hypotonic (free water) and hypertonic fluids (fruit juices) should be avoided because of the potential of increasing the stoma and stool output.[31]

Antidiarrheal Medications

Many patients with SBS rely on a high dose of antidiarrheal medications to control diarrhea and stoma output long-term. These medications, which reduce gut motility and prolong the transit of nutrients and fluids, may improve nutrient and fluid absorption.[32] Adjustments in antidiarrheal medications are often needed to minimize the diarrhea as a result of recommended increases in oral intake before any attempt at PN weaning. Commonly used antidiarrheal medications include loperamide, diphenoxylate-atropine, tincture of opium, and codeine.[33] Antidiarrheal medications should be taken within 30 to 60 minutes before meals to achieve their maximum effect.

They should be taken around the clock in most cases. Higher doses of those medications may be required because patients may develop tolerance to them over time but also because of medication malabsorption. Clonidine, an α_2-receptor agonist, has been found to reduce stool volumes (reduced fecal water and sodium losses) successfully in patients with SBS with and without colon.[34,35] Clonidine reduces gastrointestinal (GI) secretions and should be considered during the optimization process for those patients who exhibit severe diarrhea. Octreotide, a somatostatin analogue, has been shown to be effective in reducing high stoma output in patients with SBS with end-jejunostomy by reducing secretions and fluid losses.[36,37] In a small open-label trial, long-acting octreotide depot (20 mg intramuscularly) administration was associated with a significant reduction in stool losses and requirements for IV fluids and electrolytes.[38] The administration of octreotide, therefore, can offer solution for patients with SBS who are refractory to conventional therapy and who suffer from chronic dehydration and massive losses of fluids and electrolytes. However, no data are available on the effects of long-term therapy with octreotide. There is a concern about octreotide use because of risk of gallstone formation from decreased biliary tract motility. Octreotide has been also shown to impair intestinal regeneration and the adaptive response to intestinal resection by inhibition of enterocyte migration and proliferation, and increased apoptosis in animal studies.[39,40] Antibiotics should be used in the appropriate clinical scenario for suspected cases of bacterial overgrowth–related diarrhea.[41]

AGENTS PROMOTING PARENTERAL NUTRITION WEANING

Although traditional treatment strategies for SBS-IF were focused on reducing malabsorption-related losses through diet modification, ORS, and antidiarrhea/antisecretory agents, a novel targeted therapy was needed to augment the functional gut capacity of the remnant bowel and to allow for a significant reduction in PN dependence. Two intestinotrophic agents, recombinant GH and teduglutide, a GLP-2 analogue, have been approved for the PS weaning process for patients with SBS-IF in the United States.

Growth Hormone

Enhanced intestinal adaptation and nutrient absorption have been found using a GH in the SBS model, in vitro and in animal studies.[42,43] Beneficial effects of a GH include the promotion of a crypt cell proliferation and mucosal growth, and the proliferation of mesenchymal cell. Clinical studies suggested that GH, in combination with a specialized diet and glutamine, may facilitate PS weaning for patients with SBS-IF. In a study by Byrne and colleagues,[9] 47 patients (most with a colon in-continuity) received a combination of GH, oral glutamine, and an optimized diet for 3 weeks in a controlled inpatient setting. After 3 weeks of GH therapy, patients continued on their program of glutamine and a modified diet. Forty percent of patients were fully weaned from PN and another 50% of the group had clinically significant reductions in PN volumes in the follow-up for the maximum of 5 years.[44] However, the question was raised of whether or not the results could be replicated in an ambulatory setting and modified by the patient selection, optimization of the diet and medications, close monitoring, and counseling. The study by Zhu and colleagues[11] exhibited similar long-lasting effects of the GH therapy using similar regimen in an uncontrolled, prospective study. Out of 13 patients with SBS, 76%[10] of them at 1 year and 50% at 2 years were weaned from PN. In another prospective, randomized, placebo-controlled trial with recombinant analogue of GH (somatropin), 41 patients dependent on PN/IV fluid, most with colon-in-continuity, were studied in an inpatient setting for 6 weeks.[10] After 2 weeks of optimization and PN stabilization, the patients were randomized into three arms: (1) somatropin (0.10 mg/kg/d subcutaneously) with glutamine, (2) somatropin without glutamine, and (3) placebo (glutamine only) for 4 weeks. At the end of the study, both groups treated with GH achieved a significant reduction in PN requirements. In that study, the extent of PN reduction was the greatest in patients with SBS who received a combination of somatropin and glutamine. Somatropin, under brand name Zorptive (Merck Serono, Darmstadt, Germany), was approved in the United States for a short-term (4 weeks) therapy (0.1 mg/kg subcutaneous injections once daily to a maximum dose 8 mg per therapy) for the PS weaning in patients with SBS-IF in 2003.[45] Somatropin has not been widely accepted in clinical practice because of adverse effects and concerns about its efficacy. Randomized controlled studies of nutrient balance have shown conflicting results with respect to nutrient and fluid absorption in humans.[46–49]

GH actually does help retain fluid, which is important, not from enhanced gut absorption, but rather because of enhanced renal tubular reabsorption of sodium. GH-containing regimen has not been approved for PS weaning in Europe based on insufficient data to support its use.[50]

Teduglutide

GLP-2 is secreted from L-cells of ileum and a proximal colon in response to luminal nutrients. Patients with SBS after major distal small bowel and colon resection are lacking GLP-2. In animal studies, GLP-2 was found to enhance intestinal adaptation by inducing epithelial proliferation of the small and large intestine and stimulation of crypt cell proliferation, inhibiting enterocyte apoptosis, increasing blood flow to the gut mucosa, and by inhibiting gut motility.[51,52] These beneficial effects of GLP-2 were confirmed in a small, open-label trial of eight patients with SBS by showing an increase in energy absorption, a decrease in fecal wet weight, and a nonsignificant trend toward increasing jejunal villus height and crypt depth with GLP-2 twice daily.[53] In an open label trial of 16 patients with SBS, teduglutide, a recombinant GLP-2 analogue, was found to be safe, well-tolerated, and associated with a significant increase in intestinal wet weight absorption.[54] A sustained rise in plasma citrulline levels was observed in patients with SBS-IF who received teduglutide likely reflecting an increase in enterocyte mass and gut absorptive capacity.[55] To address the effects of teduglutide on PN/IV volume reduction and full weaning, all randomized and retrospective studies are reviewed.

Randomized trials

Teduglutide was studied further in two phase 3 randomized, double-blind, placebo-controlled trials. In the first trial, 83 patients with SBS were enrolled into three treatment arms (group 1, teduglutide at dose 0.05 mg/kg/d subcutaneously daily; group 2, teduglutide at 0.10 mg/kg/d; and the placebo group) and received therapy for 6 months after an optimization period.[12] The primary end point of the study was determined based on expert opinions, and it was defined as greater than or equal to 20% weekly PN/IV volume reduction by Week 20 and maintained at Week 24. Only the lower dose of teduglutide was associated with a significant reduction in weekly PN/IV volumes (teduglutide 0.05 mg/kg/d vs placebo: 46% vs 6%). Three patients were weaned from PN/IV by the end of the trial. In the extension trial of additional 28 weeks of teduglutide therapy, 68% of patients in the lower dose teduglutide group achieved greater than or equal to 20% reduction in weekly PN volume, and 68% of them had a reduction of 1 or more days off PN at the end of the study.[14] The patients who received the lower dose of teduglutide had sustained reduction in PS volume by 4.9 L/wk. PN/IV was fully weaned in four patients.

In the second study (STEPS), teduglutide at dose 0.05 mg/kg/d administered for 6 months was compared with a placebo in 86 patients with SBS with PN/IV dependency.[13] All patients who entered the study were at least 1 year from last bowel resection, and they received PN/IV infusions for more than 12 months, and at least three times a week. Weekly PS volume reduction ($\geq$20%) was achieved in 63% of patients in teduglutide group versus 30% patients in placebo group ($P = .02$). Teduglutide was superior to the placebo in the mean absolute weekly PN volume reduction (4.4 L vs 2.3 L; $P = .05$). Fifty-four percent of patients given teduglutide had reduced at least 1 PN/IV infusion day per week compared with 23% patients in the placebo group. At the end of the study, none of subjects were fully weaned from PN/IV. The significant difference in PN/IV volume reduction was observed after 8 weeks of teduglutide therapy. In the STEPS study, a more aggressive PN/IV weaning protocol was implemented, allowing for higher PS volume reductions (10%–30% vs 10%) at 2-week intervals, and the volume adjustments were started earlier (at Week 2 vs at Week 4), when compared with the initial trial.

In a 2-year extension study (STEPS-2), which included some patients from the placebo arm of the STEPS trial, 65 (74%) patients completed the study.[15] In 30 patients who completed 30 months of teduglutide therapy, a mean absolute volume reduction by 7.6 L/wk was seen, and also 70% of them eliminated at least 1 PN/IV infusion day per week. Thirteen patients achieved full enteral autonomy. A total of 15 out of the 134 (11%) patients who had received teduglutide in both phase 3 studies and their extensions were fully weaned from PN/IV.[56] Most of the patients who were able to discontinue PN had a portion of colon-in-continuity and/or had lower baseline PN/IV requirements ($\leq$6 L/wk). Because of the small number of patients who achieved weaning from PN/IV, a reliable analysis of predictive factors for weaning was impossible. In a 1-year, open-label extension study (STEPS-3) of 27 patients who previously completed the STEPS-2 trial, patients who received teduglutide for less than or equal to 36, or 42 months, had a mean PS volume reduction from baseline of 3.9 L/wk (48%) and 9.8 L/wk (50%) at the end of the trial, respectively.[57] Two patients achieved PS independence at the end of the study. In addition, two other patients who were weaned from PN/IV in the STEPS-2 maintained enteral autonomy throughout the STEPS-3 trial. In a post hoc analysis of a phase 3 placebo-controlled study (85 patients) performed to identify patient characteristics, in whom teduglutide therapy had the largest effects on parenteral support volume response, teduglutide had the greatest effect on absolute parenteral support volume reduction in the group of patients with jejunostomy/ileostomy (reduction of 919 mL/d), when compared with teduglutide-treated patients with 50% or more colon-in-continuity (reduction of 355 mL/d; $P = .006$), or the placebo (reduction of 340 mL/d; $P = .011$).[58] To summarize the phase 3 clinical studies, teduglutide therapy was associated with a sustained reduction in PS volume and the number of days off PS. However, complete weaning from PN/IV was achieved in less than 15% of patients with SBS-IF.

Retrospective studies

Teduglutide was approved for clinical use as Gattex (NPS, Bedminster, NJ) in the United States in December 2012. The drug has been also approved as Revestive (Nycomed, Zurich, Switzerland) in Europe in the same year. Since its approval for clinical use, a few retrospective studies have been published to address the effects of teduglutide on PN/IV weaning in a "real-life clinical setting" outside of controlled trials.

In a retrospective analysis of 18 patients with SBS who were treated with teduglutide, significant PN/IV volume reductions were observed in 16 patients.[59] Eleven (61%) patients achieved full enteral autonomy at a median time of 10 months (range, 3–36 months). Ten of 11 (91%) patients who achieved enteral autonomy had a colon in continuity. In another study including 14 patients with SBS-IF (nine with a colon in continuity) treated with teduglutide up to 2 years, a significant PN/IV volume reduction was achieved by 54.5% of patients at 1 year, and by 71.3% of them beyond 1 year of therapy.[60] A greater PN/IV volume reduction was observed in patients with a colon in continuity. Only two patients were weaned from PN/IV after 48 weeks of therapy. In a retrospective single-center study, 27 patients with SBS were treated with teduglutide up to 2 years.[61] A clinically significant reduction in PN/IV volume was observed in 79%[15] of patients up to 45 weeks of teduglutide therapy and 45% of those who were treated for 2 years. PN was weaned fully in 21% (4/19) of patients at the end of follow-up. In a retrospective cohort study of six patients with SBS (colon present, three; stoma, three; mean PS volume needs, 7.7 L/wk) subsequently treated with teduglutide for 24 to 36 months, all patients achieved 20% or more weekly PN/IV volume reduction within 6 months of therapy.[62] All patients were eventually weaned from PN/IV. Patients with a colon in continuity and lower weekly PS volume requirements were weaned from PN/IV sooner than those patients with stomas and higher PN/IV volume needs. In a retrospective cohort study, 13 patients with SBS (five colon in continuity, all with Crohn disease, eight [62%] on immunosuppression) received teduglutide for a median of 1 year.[63] Before the teduglutide therapy, all patients required IV fluids with a median volume 9 L/wk. With the teduglutide treatment, IV fluid requirement decreased by 3.1 L/wk. Out of nine (69%) patients who received PN, only one patient (7.7%) was on PN at the end of follow-up. Parenteral support was reduced significantly in all patients and completely discontinued in 46% of patients.[6]

To summarize the results of all available studies, a substantial variation in response (PN/IV volume reduction/weaning) to teduglutide therapy has been demonstrated among patients with SBS-IF. The number of patients fully weaned from PN/IV was much higher in the retrospective studies (20%–61%) versus phase 3 clinical trials (<15%). The difference between the PS weaning approach and patient selection may have an impact on the rate of weaning from PN/IV between both types of studies. The results of the studies suggest that teduglutide can be used for PN/IV reduction and weaning in most anatomically and clinically heterogeneous patients with SBS-IF. The response to teduglutide therapy requires a variable time frame and complete weaning from PN/IV may take months and potentially more than 2 years.[64]

Adverse effects of teduglutide

The limitations of teduglutide therapy have to be acknowledged. Common adverse effects of teduglutide include abdominal pain (34%), stoma enlargement if stoma present (33%), nausea (19%), abdominal distention (16%), injection site reactions (25%), fluid overload (14%), and bowel obstruction (11%).[13,65] Special attention should be paid to the possibility of the coexisting conditions that may contribute to the previously mentioned symptoms, such as active Crohn disease, intestinal stricture, or bacterial overgrowth. Clinicians must be prepared to manage the adverse effects during PN weaning with teduglutide, and premature drug discontinuation should be avoided (Table 2). Stoma enlargement is a result of the direct effect of teduglutide on intestinal mucosa, and this trend has been observed with small bowel stoma and colostomy.[13,59,62] Therefore, no dose reduction or discontinuation of teduglutide is needed. Common GI adverse effects (abdominal discomfort and pain, bloating, distention) are expected to dissipate over time with a continuation of teduglutide therapy. However, a

Table 2
Management of common adverse effects of teduglutide during reduction of parenteral support

Adverse Effect	Intervention
Stoma swelling/enlargement	No intervention or dose-reduction temporary May need stoma appliance adjustment or change
Abdominal pain/bloating	Consider teduglutide dose reduction Exclude other conditions: obstruction, SIBO If SIBO, treat with antibiotics Consider surgical or endoscopic intervention if mechanical obstruction and patient is a candidate for intervention Consider antibloat medications and probiotics
Bowel obstruction	Consider teduglutide discontinuation if chronic obstruction Stop teduglutide if mechanical obstruction identified Temporary teduglutide discontinuation Consider surgery if patient is a surgical candidate to correct obstruction If obstruction resolved/mechanical obstruction corrected restart therapy
CHF/fluid overload	PN/IV fluid reduction Consider diuretics Reduce temporary teduglutide dose or temporary discontinuation until condition resolved
Injection reaction	Consider dose reduction
Increased absorption of concomitant oral medications	Reduce concomitant oral medication dose Consider close frequent monitoring if blood levels for monitoring are available
Colon polyps	Colonoscopy at appropriate intervals

Abbreviations: CHF, congestive heart failure; SIBO, small intestinal bacterial overgrowth.

dose reduction or temporary discontinuation of teduglutide may be needed. Patients who have heart and/or renal disease and who are treated with teduglutide are at risk for fluid overload and congestive heart failure. Therefore, a rapid response and reduction in PS volume may be necessary to prevent congestive heart failure instead of an unnecessary discontinuation of teduglutide therapy. Another potential problem that clinicians may account for during teduglutide therapy is concomitant drug-related toxicity and adverse effects as a result of their increased intestinal absorption. This applies especially to medications with a narrow therapeutic index, such as warfarin, sedatives, and opioids.[66] Therefore, appropriate monitoring and dose adjustments of concomitant medications may be necessary to avoid those issues in a clinical setting.

Precautions and limitations
Because of the trophic nature of teduglutide, there is great concern regarding its potential for initiation and acceleration of tumor growth in the intestinal tract. Although

GLP-2 treatment with a preinduced cancer showed potential to promote growth of existing neoplasia in animals, no clear evidence exists to confirm this neoplastic effect of teduglutide in humans.[67] A recent systematic review of the potential risk of intestinal neoplasia in patients receiving treatment with GLP-2 up to 30 months without preexisting cancer did not reveal an increased risk of neoplasia.[68] However, because of the small number of patients, a conclusion regarding long-term risk of teduglutide-induced neoplasia cannot be reached. Teduglutide therapy is contraindicated in patients with active GI cancer or patients at high risk for GI cancer (eg, familial adenomatous polyposis). Potential risks and benefits need to be weighed before prescribing this therapy to patients with non-GI malignancies, and an oncologist should be involved in the decision-making process. Colon polyps have been found on a surveillance colonoscopy during teduglutide therapy.[13] A colonoscopy with removal of colon polyps should be performed within 6 months before the initiation of teduglutide therapy. Subsequent colonoscopy is recommended at the end of 1 year of teduglutide therapy and then at 5-year intervals or more often based on polyp detection. De novo formation of duodenal polyps (hematomatous) was reported in a patient who was treated with teduglutide for more than 1 year.[69] Upper GI tract surveillance for neoplasia has not been standardized; however, some medical centers (verbal communication) perform routine upper endoscopies during teduglutide therapy. At present, no recommendations have been published on endoscopic surveillance of the upper GI tract. The risk of neoplasia is one of major concerns for patients to decline teduglutide therapy.

Administration
Teduglutide at a dose of 0.05 mg/kg/d is administered subcutaneously once a day. Patients with a creatinine clearance of less than 50 mL/min require a 50% dose reduction. Patient compliance with daily injections is important during the PN weaning process. Patients should stay on the teduglutide therapy long-term in cases of a good response to the therapy. In a study by Compher and colleagues,[70] teduglutide discontinuation (at the end of clinical trial) was associated with a need to restart PN/IV in most patients, especially those with high PN/IV volume requirements at baseline. The results of this study confirm a short-lasting effect of teduglutide therapy on gut mucosa. Antiteduglutide antibodies have been detected in the blood of patients treated with teduglutide.[15] These antibodies are most likely nonneutralizing because their presence has not been associated with a negative effect on PS volume reduction. The data on the discontinuation rate of teduglutide therapy because of the lack of efficacy or adverse effects are limited. Criteria for the discontinuation of teduglutide therapy have not been well defined. Although teduglutide therapy is well-tolerated, efficacy and safety should be closely monitored on an ongoing basis in all patients.

Cost and availability
The estimated annual cost of teduglutide therapy is approximately $300,000.[71] The cost is covered by most insurance plans in the United States. Although teduglutide therapy is available for patients with SBS-IF in the United States and a few European countries, it is not wildly available elsewhere. Unfortunately, clinicians in many countries have no opportunity to use this therapy for their patients with SBS-IF because of governmental restrictions. The high cost of teduglutide therapy limits its use across the globe. Because of the economic burden associated with teduglutide therapy, identification of predictive markers for clinical response and patient selection to this regimen is critically important.

Novel GLP-2 Agents in Development

The last few years have witnessed the development of new GLP-2 analogues. Two long-acting GLP-2 analogues, apraglutide (Therachon, Basel, Switzerland) and glepaglutide (Zealand Pharma, Glostrup, Denmark), are currently in preclinical studies. These agents may be advantageous because of the need for less frequent injections and the probability of higher efficacy on PN/IV weaning for patients with SBS-IF. Recently, apraglutide was shown to stimulate linear intestinal growth in the animal model of SBS without ileum.[72] In addition, the combination of GLP-1 and GLP-2 (potent coagonists) was also recently investigated with regard to its potential benefits over the existing monotherapy for SBS. In an animal SBS model, GLP-1/GLP-2 coagonists showed a significant impact on gut adaptation by indicating a marked increase in intestinal volume and a mucosal surface area, and also positive effects on body weight and gastric emptying.[73] These drugs in the pipeline may potentially offer additional benefits in PN volume reduction in SBS-IF in the near future.

PARENTERAL NUTRITION WEANING
Methods and Settings

There is a shortfall of published guidelines about the most appropriate strategy for achieving successful weaning from parenteral support. General options of PN weaning are shown in **Table 3**. Clinicians may choose between two methods of gradual reduction of PN/IV volume. The first method involves gradually reducing the number of administration days, and the second involves reducing PN volume infused each day by certain percentage. The second method carries a lower risk of dehydration, and therefore may be safer. However, patients often prefer a reduction in days of PN/IV because of convenience. In some settings, PN is substituted first by IV hydration, if the primary issue is excessive fluid losses but body weight is maintained, or the patient suffers from recurrent sepsis from central line–associated bloodstream infections. This approach, a transition from PN to IV fluids, is also considered during PN weaning with teduglutide therapy in patients with recurrent sepsis. Transitioning from PN to IV fluids may be attempted either before or during the weaning process with teduglutide therapy. PN/IV weaning process is done with or without a trophic agent. In most cases, the PN/IV weaning using the standard approach should be attempted first (**Fig. 1**). Because teduglutide therapy has a major impact on facilitating the PN weaning, teduglutide-based weaning strategy should be considered after standard measures have failed. In addition, the weaning process is accomplished in the inpatient or outpatient settings, depending on patient's clinical status and available resources. In stable patients with SBS who exhibit favorable factors for independence from PN, the weaning process should be initiated in early stages of SBS-IF. In patients with unfavorable prognostic factors, attempts of PS weaning should be delayed (after

---

Table 3
General approach to weaning from parenteral support (methods, adjuvant regimens facilitating weaning, and setting)

Method	Adjuvant Trophic Agent	Combined with Enteral Nutrition Support	Settings
Gradual reduction of PN volume	No without teduglutide	No	Inpatient
Reduction of days off PN/IV	Yes with teduglutide	Yes	Outpatient

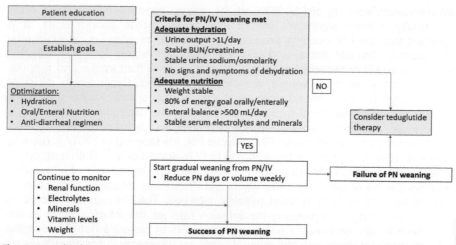

Fig. 1. Standard approach to parenteral support weaning. BUN, blood urea nitrogen.

more than 1 year from surgery, awaiting completion of intestinal adaptation), or consideration should be given to the teduglutide-based strategy (**Fig. 2**). The PN weaning process can also be facilitated by using EN in addition to the oral diet. EN promotes intestinal adaptation and has been beneficial for successful weaning from PN/IV in select patients.

Parenteral Nutrition Weaning in Inpatient Settings

In the early postoperative period, patients with SBS should receive PN, at least in the first 7 to 10 days, to ensure proper nutrition and hydration until hemodynamic stability is achieved. This is followed by a transition, whenever possible, to EN and/or an oral diet.[16] The composition and volume of the formulation and the number of PN infusions should be adjusted to each patient's individual needs. Before the

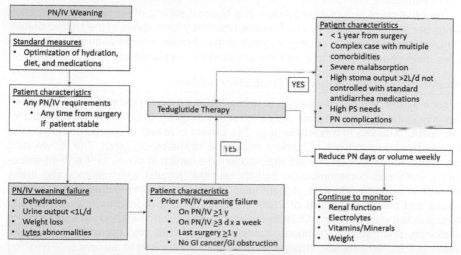

Fig. 2. When to initiate teduglutide therapy as part of PN/IV weaning strategy.

discontinuation/weaning of PN, 80% of the energy needs must be taken orally or enterally, without significant weight loss or electrolyte abnormalities. It is important that the PN weaning process should occur as soon as possible after the patient is clinically stable, and positive prognostic factors for PN/IV weaning are identified. PN/IV reduction is safely attempted while fluid intake and outputs, and electrolytes and body weight, are closely monitored. Cyclic PN/IV infusions (eg, overnight for 8–16 hours) encourage oral or/and enteral intake during the day. The length of the PN/IV cycle should be adjusted depending on the oral or enteral intake and the patient's tolerance of any higher rate of parenteral infusion. After the change from continuous PN to cyclic PN, the tapering of PN/IV is done by volume reduction, days off, or transitioning to IV hydration only.[74] Both methods of gradual reduction of PN/IV are used in hospital setting. The number of administration days can be reduced by 1 per week, but PN volume infused per day can be reduced by 10% to 30% in short (weekly) intervals. The PN regimen should be adjusted accordingly, decreasing the infusion rate (or the infusion time) as the oral/enteral intake increases. Periodic assessments of patient's nutritional status and hydration and electrolyte and mineral levels are necessary during the PN weaning process. There are multiple benefits of enteral intake, including promotion of intestinal adaptation. In cases of difficulty with PN weaning, EN should be considered. EN should be started gradually in a hemodynamically stable patient after bowel function is restored and stool output is less than 2 L/d. However, in case of high stoma/stool output greater than 2 L/d, oral or enteral intake could aggravate the diarrhea and could lead to dehydration and electrolyte imbalance. Strategies aimed to promote the patient's normal appetite and to encourage an increase in oral/enteral intake are important so that reliance on the PN is gradually reduced. During transitional feeding, PN is converted to enteral or oral nutrition with a subsequent discontinuation of PN. This transition may take a few days, or several weeks. Patients should demonstrate the ability to maintain weight, hydration, electrolytes, and nutrient balance before PN/IV discontinuation. Before trials with teduglutide, PN weaning has been conducted often in inpatient settings. This approach has allowed for close monitoring, diet, and ORS reinforcement, at the same time allowing for a more rapid weaning process when compared with alternative ambulatory settings.

The initiation of teduglutide therapy in a hospital setting often presents as a challenge because the drug is not on hospital pharmacy formularies in the United States. Patients who are already undergoing teduglutide therapy should continue daily injections during hospitalization, if no contraindications are identified.

Parenteral Nutrition Weaning in Ambulatory Settings

In general, the process of weaning of home PN/IV solution is different from PN weaning in hospital settings. Patient desire to reduce or discontinue PN/IV is important for successful weaning in a home setting. The patient is asked to measure urine output frequently and keep track of nutrient intake and stoma/stool output. The PS weaning process also requires dedicated practitioner time, which is set up for frequent ambulatory visits and communication (telephone calls, emails) with patients and home parenteral support agencies, for frequent review of urine measurements and oral intake and the management of PN/IV adjustments and monitoring/management of teduglutide therapy, if used. Multidisciplinary team approach is often needed including clinicians, pharmacists, dietitians, home visiting nurses, and home care agencies. Well-coordinated care and strong communication is required to achieve safe weaning from PN. In the best scenario, all patients with SBS-IF should be referred to centers with expertise in intestinal rehabilitation for evaluation and management of PN weaning, especially for the stabilization and initiation of weaning. If the visit to a specialized center is not feasible for a patient, a local practitioner should establish a connection with an expert in intestinal rehabilitation for timely communication, if needed. The following sections are dedicated to the weaning from PN/IV in an ambulatory setting.

Energy and fluid intake targets should be established to maintain patient body weight before the initiation of the weaning process. Energy goals should be determined by calculating resting energy expenditure combined with the activity level and malabsorption factors. Realistic target body weight should be established that enables optimal functioning. The PN weaning process should be attempted after the diet, oral hydration, and drug regimen are optimized. The patient should be clinically stable before the onset of the weaning process and should not require frequent adjustments in PS volume, calories, and/or electrolytes. There should be no need for dose changes in antidiarrheal medications and other drug therapies for any active disease. Patient should not be awaiting any type of surgery. Daily caloric intake should be steady before an attempt of reducing PN/IV.

Teduglutide plays an important role in the PN/IV weaning after unsuccessful attempts to wean patients off PN with standard measures. Teduglutide allows for the reduction in PN/IV volumes and calories, and eventually for the full weaning from PN/IV. However, the patient should be made aware that complete PN weaning may not be achieved with this therapy. To achieve successful weaning with teduglutide, several criteria must be met (**Box 3**).

Timing of Parenteral Nutrition Weaning with Teduglutide

Traditionally, in patients with SBS-IF at high risk for PN dependence, an attempt of weaning was often conducted after the intestinal adaptation process was complete

---

Box 3
When to consider teduglutide therapy in a patient with SBS-IF during PN/IV weaning

- Clinically stable and well-nourished patient
- Optimized diet and hydration therapy
- Motivated patient with a desire to discontinue the parenteral support
- Patient agreeable to close monitoring of response to therapy (blood work, weight, urine output measurements, diet diary)
- Prior compliance with other therapies and follow-up visits
- Failure of PN/IV weaning with diet and hydration optimization and maximum of antidiarrheal regimen
  - PN/IV fluids >3 times per week
  - PN duration >1 year
  - Other considerations:
    - PN/IV fluids <1 year and
      - Serious PN complications ≥2 septic episodes or central access lost
      - Uncontrolled stool or stoma output with conventional antidiarrheal agents and high demand for IV fluids and nutrients
- No contraindication
  - No active bowel stricture, mechanical obstruction, active Crohn disease
  - No active GI cancer
  - If active or prior non-GI cancer consider therapy based on risk versus benefit ratio assessment after consultation with oncologist

(1–2 years) to increase the probability of successful weaning from PN/IV. In phase 3 clinical trials, all patients with SBS-IF enrolled in teduglutide therapy were at least 1 year from last surgery to guarantee clinical stability and completion of the intestinal adaptation process, and they were dependent on PN/IV for more than 1 year.[13] This resulted in routine consideration of teduglutide therapy only after 1 year of PN/IV dependence. However, the earliest time to introduce teduglutide therapy for PN/IV weaning has not been articulated by any scientific evidence or experts. Nevertheless, with the advent of teduglutide, an attempt of PN weaning could be probably considered much sooner (within 1 year from the last surgery/onset of SBS and PN dependence <1 year). There seems to be a concern whether or not early treatment with teduglutide may alter the natural process of intestinal adaptation in a negative way. Another thought process would suggest that teduglutide may induce super-hyperadaptation and may accelerate the intestinal adaptation. Teduglutide may also increase the absorption of nutrients and fluids in addition to potentially allowing for early PN/IV elimination.

Most likely, teduglutide therapy could be introduced at a much earlier stage of IF (possibly 3–6 months after surgery) in appropriate settings (clinically stable patient) to initiate the PN/IV weaning process. Other patients who would possibly benefit from early teduglutide therapy include those with severe malnutrition/massive fluid losses poorly controlled with parenteral therapy and PN-related complications (recurrent central line–associated bloodstream infections, or central access issues). Although this approach is beyond current practice standards for the use of teduglutide, the initiation of this therapy much sooner would offer clear benefits, including earlier stabilization of the patient and the weaning from PN/IV much earlier, therefore avoiding PN-related complications. In a clinical practice study, the PN/IV weaning process with teduglutide was introduced in a few patients less than a year after the initiation of parenteral support in patients with SBS-IF because of their poor health status, severe malnutrition, and high demand for an earlier intervention.[61] Further studies are needed to evaluate this concept.

Patient Selection for Parenteral Nutrition Weaning with Teduglutide

In cases of unsuccessful PN weaning using a standard approach, a decision should be made if the patient is a good candidate for teduglutide therapy. Most patients with SBS dependent on PN/IV are suitable for teduglutide therapy (see **Box 3**). Currently, the presence of a colon and the length of the remaining small bowel, and underlying disease, duration of PN dependence, and PN volume requirement do not influence the selection of candidates for teduglutide therapy. At present, no clear criteria exist to predict which patients achieve full weaning from PN/IV with teduglutide therapy. Perhaps, the patients with a colon in continuity, lower PN/IV volume requirements, and lower number of PN/IV days have a much higher probability of full PN/IV weaning.[56,59] A high compliance with teduglutide therapy and optimization process is critical for successful weaning.

A higher probability of greater absolute volume reduction PN/IV was observed in patients with end-jejunostomy and higher volume needs.[58,64] This finding is a result of a more beneficial effect of teduglutide in patients who are unable to produce GLP-2 (after distal small bowel and colon resection). Patients without colon or shorter length of the colon and patients with stoma and PN/IV needs greater than 6 L/d were found to have higher probability of early response (significant volume reduction) within 6 months.[64] Patients with SBS-IF with current obstructive symptoms or active GI malignancy must be excluded from teduglutide therapy. In cases of prior or current non-GI cancer, a clinician must decide if teduglutide therapy is appropriate based on the risk-benefit ratio and an oncologist input. Although patients should be in optimal nutritional and fluid balance before PN weaning, patients with SBS-IF with high fluid and nutrient demands may also be considered for teduglutide therapy.

PARENTERAL NUTRITION WEANING

After the optimization process, gradual PN reductions should be made by either decreasing the days/frequency of PN infusions per week or by a partial reduction of the PN volumes infused daily. Subsequent PN/IV reductions are based on tolerance determined by hydration status, urine output, electrolytes, and weight changes and symptoms.[33] Several criteria should be met before any adjustments in parenteral support.[16] Daily fluid goal ought to be met to prevent dehydration. Hydration status should be monitored closely. Hydration status and PS reduction feasibility should be assessed by measurement of urine output. The most reliable marker of adequate hydration is urine output between 1 and 2 L/d. PN/IV volume reduction should be considered only when urine output exceeds 1 L/d and is at least 0.5 mL/kg/h on PN/IV-free days, or after prior volume reduction. Although frequent measurements of urine output are challenging for the patient, this method provides most critical information on patient's hydration status to guide the PN weaning process. The patient should maintain positive enteral fluid balance (oral fluid intake minus stool output) by at least 500 mL/d. Serum creatinine, blood urea nitrogen, urine sodium, and osmolarity can also be used as surrogate marker of hydration. Urinary sodium concentration should be more than 20 mEq/L.

An algorithm for PN/IV volume reduction that was implemented in the clinical trials with teduglutide can be applied to facilitate PN weaning with or without teduglutide (**Fig. 3**).

Gradual PN/IV reductions (10%–30% of volume) seem to be safe and may provide a higher probability for weaning. Urine daily volume and weight should be monitored before and after each PN/IV adjustment. Patients often prefer a reduction in PN days, but this approach may carry a higher risk of dehydration. It seems reasonable to start first with gradual volume reductions and later to switch the process to days off PN/IV. An optimal interval for making PN reductions has not been well defined. In the outpatient setting, volume reductions at 1- to 2-week intervals seem to be safe and allow patient's body adjustment to PN/IV changes. Perhaps, the intervals for PN adjustments should be individualized for each patient and tailored to clinical response and patient's preference. After PN infusions are reduced to less than 3 days per week, an attempt of full PN discontinuation is reasonable. However, the decision has to be individualized based on the PN volume requirement, urine output, and renal function.

In addition, daily energy target should be met by oral and/or enteral intake. The body weight should be stable with less than a 1.5-kg drop in weight between PN/IV reductions. Food and fluid charts are beneficial to record the patient's oral and enteral intake. Energy, protein, and fluid intakes should be monitored by the dietitian to ensure that nutritional goals are met by oral intake. Some patients, who are mainly energy dependent, may tolerate significant calories and protein reduction in the PN, but their fluid volume has to be sustained for adequate hydration.

Serum electrolyte and mineral levels should be stable during the weaning process. Laboratory studies (electrolytes, renal function) need to be monitored weekly or after each PN adjustment during the weaning process. Measurements of serum citrulline have been tested in clinical trials; however, there are no data to support the use serum

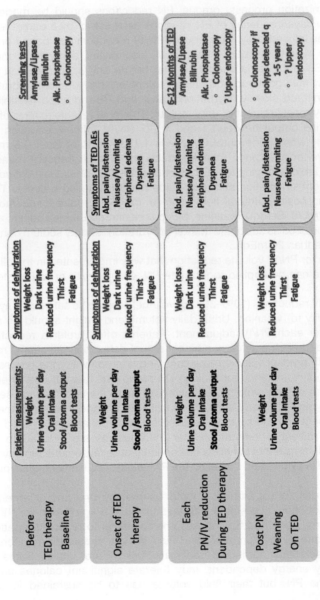

Fig. 3. Monitoring during teduglutide-based PN/IV weaning. Abd, abdominal; AE, adverse event; TED, teduglutide.

citrulline as a predictor of response to teduglutide therapy and a success of PN weaning. During PN weaning, transition from parenteral to oral supplementation of vitamin and trace elements and minerals should be done to ensure that the normal blood levels are maintained.

Clinical decisions whether to start teduglutide therapy or not should be guided by treatment goals, physician judgment, and patient preferences. Patients on teduglutide therapy need additional monitoring (**Fig. 4**) and management of its adverse effects, if they should arise. Close monitoring (office visits every 4 weeks, telephone contacts if significant changes in stool/stoma output or body weight) is necessary to confirm patient compliance with the weaning strategy and response to teduglutide therapy. Diet modifications and the use of ORS and compliance with antidiarrheal regimen should be reinforced during each visit. Clinical examination at the office or during home nursing visits should be focused on signs suggestive of dehydration or fluid overload. The symptom of shortness of breath requires immediate attention to the possibility of fluid overload and congestive heart failure. If the patient shows signs of suboptimal hydration and/or poor nutritional status following PN/IV volume reduction, critical consideration should be given to increasing or restarting PN/IV.

Some reimbursement issues may arise with any major reduction in the number of PN infusions or calories, or a switch to the exclusive IV hydration. Parenteral support coverage may be denied by insurance plans if specified caloric requirements or the number of days per week of PN are not met.[74]

WEANING PARENTERAL NUTRITION IN COMBINATION WITH ENTERAL NUTRITION SUPPORT

EN, if tolerated, may help to achieve successful PN weaning. Continuous tube feeding, either alone or in combination with oral nutrition, allows for persistent luminal stimulation and improved macronutrient absorption.[75,76] Joly and colleagues[77] have shown that continuous tube feeding (1000 kcal/d), exclusively or in conjunction with oral nutrition during postoperative period (>3 months), was associated with a significant increase in absorption of lipids, proteins, and energy when compared with oral feeding

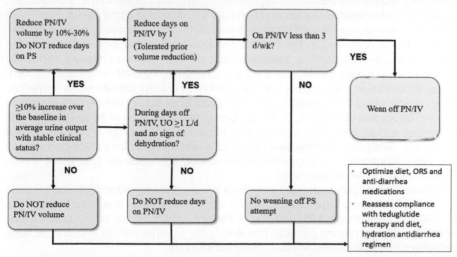

Fig. 4. PN/IV weaning protocol with use of teduglutide based on urine output. UO, urine output.

only. If patients cannot achieve energy goals with oral intake and have sufficient length of small bowel, supplemental tube feeding should be strongly considered. Cyclic nocturnal tube feeding is preferred. The administration of enteral feeding at a slow rate may improve nutrient absorption and reduce the risk of diarrhea. Polymeric formulas are preferred, because they are cheaper, less hyperosmolar, offer greater impact on intestinal adaptation, and are well-tolerated.[78,79] Semi or elemental formulas may be necessary to facilitate better nutrient absorption in cases of intolerance to polymeric formulas (bloating, diarrhea). After a trial of nasoenteric tube feeding to document feeding tolerance, gastrostomy or jejunostomy tube placement may facilitate enteral feeding, when there is a sufficient length of small bowel.[80] Aggressive use of EN is not only one of the most important factors in promoting intestinal adaptation, but it also allows for the avoidance of complications associated with PN. Therefore, EN support should be considered in patients with PN-related complications.

CONSIDERATIONS AFTER PARENTERAL NUTRITION WEANING

After a complete PS weaning, patients require regular visits to confirm stable hydration and nutritional status and regular monitoring of electrolytes and trace elements and vitamin and mineral levels. Adequate oral intake and sustained hydration should be emphasized during each visit. Antidiarrheal medications should be continued and adjusted accordingly to the degree of diarrhea/stool output. Minerals, trace elements, and vitamin levels should be periodically monitored. The frequency with which each individual patient is monitored depends on the prior history of existing deficiencies. For patients successfully weaned from PN/IV, the monitoring of electrolytes and micronutrients weekly or every 2 weeks is initially recommended. Meanwhile, the interval for monitoring of vitamin and mineral levels every 3 months seems to be reasonable. If any deficiency is detected, more frequent monitoring may be needed. Less frequent monitoring is appropriate if the patient has been off PN/IV for a long time and if all levels are normal. It is also imperative to periodically (every 2 years) monitor for metabolic bone disease.

Oral micronutrients supplementation is often necessary after PN/IV weaning. Patients may require oral electrolyte supplements, typically magnesium and potassium. In addition, bicarbonate supplementation may be needed in some cases. Significant hypomagnesemia may be seen in patients with distal ileum resection because magnesium is mainly absorbed in the distal small bowel. Because oral magnesium can induce or exacerbate diarrhea, parenteral replacement may be necessary, especially if patients have severe symptomatic hypomagnesemia. Patients with a colon in continuity should be on a supplement of oral calcium to prevent oxalate stone formation. Patients after distal ileum resection are also at a higher risk for deficiencies of vitamin B_{12} and fat-soluble vitamins (A, D, and E). Oral supplementation of those vitamins may be sufficient. However, some patients may require parenteral supplementation of the previously mentioned vitamins. In addition, zinc and essential fatty acids deficiencies can arise. Monitoring and supplementation of zinc and essential fatty acids should also be taken under consideration.

Patients on teduglutide therapy may have fewer problems associated with mineral, vitamin, and electrolyte deficiencies; however, a recent study suggests further need for oral supplements post-PN weaning.[59] Patients who continue teduglutide therapy after PS weaning require periodic monitoring for adverse effects and should have surveillance colonoscopies at recommended intervals.

In patients who demonstrate suboptimal hydration or nutrition status after full PN/IV weaning, the restarting of PN/IV should be considered. Short-term parenteral support may be required during acute or prolonged illness associated with dehydration and hypermetabolism, or prolonged fasting, because patients with SBS-IF have a low nutrient and fluid reserve. Clinicians should have a low threshold to initiate PN/IV early in this setting to prevent dehydration and malnutrition.

SUMMARY

Many patients with SBS-IF require long-term PN and/or IV fluids. Regaining oral nutritional autonomy for patients with SBS-IF is associated with an improved quality of life and the future avoidance of PN-related complications. Therefore, efforts should be made to reduce or eliminate PN/IV requirements, when feasible, in all PS-dependent patients. The PN/IV weaning process is complex and requires proper patient education, motivation, establishing realistic goals, and complying with the weaning protocol. The optimization process that includes dietary modifications, adequate hydration, and medications is critical to the success of PS weaning. The emergence of teduglutide therapy has reshaped treatment approach to PN/IV weaning strategy. Teduglutide plays an important role in facilitating the PN weaning process in patients for whom standard measures have previously failed. The positive impact of teduglutide therapy on the quality of life of patients with SBS-IF may not only be the result of a reduction in parenteral support and PN-related issues, but also of the reduction in diarrhea and an improved oral intake (stemming from the reduction in diarrhea). Because of the heterogenicity of the patients with regards to bowel anatomy, PN/IV requirements, and underlying disease, the response to teduglutide-based weaning therapy may vary. The use of teduglutide adds more complexity to the PS weaning process. Health care providers must be familiar with the indications and limitations of teduglutide therapy to achieve successful and safe PN weaning. Multiteam approach is preferred because of the complexity of PN/IV weaning strategy, which requires close patient monitoring, attention to adverse effects, and concomitant PN/IV adjustments.

At present, the PN/IV weaning algorithm, which is based on monitoring the changes in urinary output, is the best guidance for safe PN/IV volume reductions. Other subjective markers, such as a patient's general condition, body weight, thirst, and stool frequency, should be considered and during PN/IV weaning. Patients should actively participate in the decision-making process regarding the rate of PN/IV reduction to ensure a safe weaning process. In addition to patient characteristics, the rate at which patients are weaned may depend on the clinician's experience with the novel treatment approach. Patients undergoing PN weaning require continuous monitoring of nutritional and fluid status and adequate vitamin and minerals supplementation throughout PN/IV and after achieving independence from PN/IV.

REFERENCES

1. O'Keefe SJ, Buchman AL, Fishbein TM, et al. Short bowel syndrome and intestinal failure: consensus definitions and overview. Clin Gastroenterol Hepatol 2006; 4:6–10.
2. Pironi L, Arends J, Bozzetti F, et al, Home Artificial Nutrition & Chronic Intestinal Failure Special Interest Group of ESPEN. ESPEN guidelines on chronic intestinal failure in adults. Clin Nutr 2016;35:247–307.
3. Ukleja A, Romano MM. Complications of parenteral nutrition. Gastroenterol Clin North Am 2007;36:23–46.
4. Lappas BM, Patel D, Kumpf V, et al. Parenteral nutrition: indications, access, and complications. Gastroenterol Clin North Am 2018;47:39–59.

5. Amiot A, Messing B, Corcos O, et al. Determinants of home parenteral nutrition dependence and survival of 268 patients with non-malignant short bowel syndrome. Clin Nutr 2013;32:368–74.

6. Scolapio JS, Savoy AD, Kaplan J, et al. Sleep patterns of cyclic parenteral nutrition, a pilot study: are there sleepless nights? JPEN J Parenter Enteral Nutr 2002; 26:214–7.

7. Pironi L, Corcos O, Forbes A, et al, ESPEN Acute and Chronic Intestinal Failure Special Interest Groups. Intestinal failure in adults: recommendations from the ESPEN expert groups. Clin Nutr 2018;37:1798–809.

8. Messing B, Crenn P, Beau P, et al. Long-term survival and parenteral nutrition dependence in adult patients with the short bowel syndrome. Gastroenterology 1999;117:1043–50.

9. Byrne TA, Persinger RL, Young LS, et al. A new treatment for patients with short-bowel syndrome: growth hormone, glutamine, and a modified diet. Ann Surg 1995;222:243–54 [discussion: 254–5].

10. Byrne TA, Wilmore DW, Iyer K, et al. Growth hormone, glutamine, and an optimal diet reduces parenteral nutrition in patients with short bowel syndrome: a prospective, randomized, placebo-controlled, double-blind clinical trial. Ann Surg 2005;242:655–61.

11. Zhu W, Li N, Ren J, et al. Rehabilitation therapy for short bowel syndrome. Chin Med J 2002;115:776–8.

12. Jeppesen PB, Gilroy R, Pertkiewicz M, et al. Randomised placebo controlled trial of teduglutide in reducing parenteral nutrition and/or intravenous fluid requirements in patients with short bowel syndrome. Gut 2011;60:902–14.

13. Jeppesen PB, Pertkiewicz M, Messing B, et al. Teduglutide reduces need for parenteral support among patients with short bowel syndrome with intestinal failure. Gastroenterology 2012;143:1473–81.

14. O'Keefe SJ, Jeppesen PB, Gilroy R, et al. Safety and efficacy of teduglutide after 52 weeks of treatment in patients with short bowel intestinal failure. Clin Gastroenterol Hepatol 2013;11:815–23.

15. Schwartz LK, O'Keefe SJ, Jeppesen PB, et al. Long-term safety and efficacy of teduglutide for the treatment of intestinal failure associated with short bowel syndrome: final results of the STEPS-2 study, a 2-year, multicenter, open-label clinical trial. Am J Gastroenterol 2013;108:S101.

16. DiBaise JK, Matarese LE, Messing B, et al. Strategies for parenteral nutrition weaning in adult patients with short bowel syndrome. J Clin Gastroenterol 2006;40(Suppl 2):S94–8.

17. Messing B, Joly F. Guidelines for management of home parenteral support in adult chronic intestinal failure patients. Gastroenterology 2006;130(2 Suppl 1): S43–51.

18. Seidner DL, Schwartz LK, Winkler MF, et al. Increased intestinal absorption in the era of teduglutide and its impact on management strategies in patients with short bowel syndrome-associated intestinal failure. JPEN J Parenter Enteral Nutr 2013; 37:201–11.

19. Tappenden KA. Intestinal adaptation following resection. JPEN J Parenter Enteral Nutr 2014;38(1 Suppl):23S–31S.

20. Byrne TA, Veglia LM, Camelio M, et al. Beyond the prescription: optimizing the diet of patients with short bowel syndrome. Nutr Clin Pract 2000;15:306–11.

21. Woolf GM, Miller C, Kurian R, et al. Diet for patients with short bowel: high fat or high carbohydrate? Gastroenterology 1983;84:823–8.

22. Jeppesen PB, Mortensen PB. The influence of a preserved colon on the absorption of medium chain fat in patients with small bowel resection. Gut 1998;43: 478–83.
23. Jeppesen PB, Fuglsang KA. Nutritional therapy in adult short bowel syndrome patients with chronic intestinal failure. Gastroenterol Clin North Am 2018;47: 61–75.
24. Hessov I, Andersson H, Isaksson B. Effects of a low-fat diet on mineral absorption in small-bowel diseas5e. Scand J Gastroenterol 1983;18:551–4.
25. Atia A, Girard-Pipau F, Hébuterne X, et al. Macronutrient absorption characteristics in humans with short bowel syndrome and jejunocolonic anastomosis: starch is the most important carbohydrate substrate, although pectin supplementation may modestly enhance short chain fatty acid production and fluid absorption. JPEN J Parenter Enteral Nutr 2011;35:229–40.
26. Nordgaard I, Hensen BS, Mortensen PB. Colon as a digestive organ in patients with short bowel. Lancet 1994;343:373–6.
27. Earnest DL, Johnson G, Williams HE, et al. Hyperoxaluria in patients with ileal resection: an abnormality in dietary oxalate absorption. Gastroenterology 1974; 66:1114–22.
28. Ukleja A, Rivas J. Cholelithiasis and nephrolithiasis. In: DiBaise J, editor. A book chapter for short bowel syndrome: practical approach to management. Florida: CRC Press,Taylor & Francis Group; 2016. p. 81–95. Chapter 7.
29. Crenn P, Morin MC, Joly F, et al. Net digestive absorption and adaptive hyperphagia in adult short bowel patients. Gut 2004;53:1279–86.
30. Matarese LE, O'Keefe SJ, Kandil HM, et al. Short bowel syndrome: clinical guidelines for nutrition management. Nutr Clin Pract 2005;20:493–502.
31. Matarese LE. Nutrition and fluid optimization for patients with short bowel syndrome. JPEN J Parenter Enteral Nutr 2013;37:161–70.
32. King RFGJ, Norton T, Hill GL. A double-blind cross over study of the effect of loperamide hydrochloride and codeine phosphate on ileostomy output. Aust N Z J Surg 1982;52:121–4.
33. Bechtold ML, McClave SA, Palmer LB, et al. The pharmacologic treatment of short bowel syndrome: new tricks and novel agents. Curr Gastroenterol Rep 2014;16:392.
34. McDoniel K, Taylor B, Huey W, et al. Use of clonidine to decrease intestinal fluid losses in patients with high-output short-bowel syndrome. JPEN J Parenter Enteral Nutr 2004;28:265–8.
35. Buchman AL, Fryer J, Wallin A, et al. Clonidine reduces diarrhea and sodium loss in patients with proximal jejunostomy: a controlled study. JPEN J Parenter Enteral Nutr 2006;30:487–91.
36. O'Keefe SJ, Peterson ME, Fleming CR. Octreotide as an adjunct to home parenteral nutrition in the management of permanent end-jejunostomy syndrome. JPEN J Parenter Enteral Nutr 1994;18:26–34.
37. O'Keefe SJ, Haymond MW, Bennet WM, et al. Long-acting somatostatin analogue therapy and protein metabolism in patients with jejunostomies. Gastroenterology 1994;107:379–88.
38. Gómez-Herrera E, Farías-Llamas OA, Gutiérrez-de la Rosa JL, et al. The role of long-acting release (LAR) depot octreotide as adjuvant management of short bowel disease. Cir 2004;72:379–86.
39. Sukhotnik I, Khateeb K, Krausz MM, et al. Sandostatin impairs postresection intestinal adaptation in a rat model of short bowel syndrome. Dig Dis Sci 2002; 47:2095–102.

40. Thompson JS. Somatostatin analogue predisposes enterocytes to apoptosis. J Gastrointest Surg 1998;2:167–73.
41. Adike A, DiBaise JK. Small intestinal bacterial overgrowth: nutritional implications, diagnosis, and management. Gastroenterol Clin North Am 2018;47:193–208.
42. Wheeler EE, Challacombe DN. The trophic action of growth hormone, insulin-like growth factor-I, and insulin on human duodenal mucosa cultured in vitro. Gut 1997;40:57–60.
43. Ziegler TR, Estívariz CF, Jonas CR, et al. Interactions between nutrients and peptide growth factors in intestinal growth, repair, and function. JPEN J Parenter Enteral Nutr 1999;23(6 Suppl):S174–83.
44. Byrne TA, Cox S, Karimbakas M, et al. Bowel rehabilitation: an alternative to long-term parenteral nutrition and intestinal transplantation for some patients with short bowel syndrome. Transplant Proc 2002;34:887–90.
45. Matarese LE, Abu-Elmagd K. Somatropin for the treatment of short bowel syndrome in adults. Expert Opin Pharmacother 2005;6:1741–50.
46. Scolapio JS, Camilleri M, Fleming CR, et al. Effect of growth hormone, glutamine, and diet on adaptation in short bowel syndrome: a randomized, controlled study. Gastroenterology 1997;113:1074–81.
47. Szkudlarek J, Jeppesen PB, Mortensen PB. Effect of high dose growth hormone with glutamine and no change in diet on intestinal absorption in short bowel patients: a randomized, double-blind, crossover, placebo-controlled study. Gut 2000;47:199–205.
48. Seguy D, Vahedi K, Kapel N, et al. Low-dose growth hormone in adult home parenteral nutrition-dependent short bowel syndrome patients: a positive study. Gastroenterology 2003;124:293–302.
49. Wales PW, Nasr A, de Silva N, et al. Human growth hormone and glutamine for patients with short bowel syndrome. Cochrane Database Syst Rev 2010;(6):CD006321.
50. Van Gossum A, Cabre E, Hébuterne X, et al. ESPEN guidelines on parenteral nutrition: gastroenterology. Clin Nutr 2009;28:415–27.
51. Drucker DJ, Erlich P, Asa SL, et al. Induction of intestinal epithelial proliferation by glucagon-like peptide 2. Proc Natl Acad Sci U S A 1996;93:7911–6.
52. Drucker DJ, Boushey RP, Wang F, et al. Biologic properties and therapeutic potential of glucagon-like peptide-2. JPEN J Parenter Enteral Nutr 1999;23(5 Suppl):S98–100.
53. Jeppesen PB, Hartmann B, Thulesen J, et al. Glucagon-like peptide 2 improves nutrient absorption and nutritional status in short-bowel patients with no colon. Gastroenterology 2001;120:806–15.
54. Jeppesen PB, Sanguinetti EL, Buchman A, et al. Teduglutide (ALX0600), a dipeptidyl peptidase IV resistant glucagon-like peptide analogue, improves intestinal function in short bowel syndrome patients. Gut 2005;54:1224–31.
55. Seidner DL, Joly F, Youssef NN. Effect of teduglutide, a glucagon-like peptide 2 analog, on citrulline levels in patients with short bowel syndrome in two phase III randomized trials. Clin Transl Gastroenterol 2015;6:e93.
56. Iyer KR, Joelsson B, Heinze H, et al. Complete enteral autonomy and independence from parenteral nutrition/intravenous support in short bowel syndrome with intestinal failure: accruing experience with teduglutide. Gastroenterology 2013;144:S169.
57. Seidner DL, Fujioka K, Boullata JI, et al. Reduction of parenteral nutrition and hydration support and safety with long-term teduglutide treatment in patients with short bowel syndrome-associated intestinal failure: STEPS-3 study. Nutr Clin Pract 2018;33:520–7.

58. Jeppesen PB, Gabe SM, Seidner DL, et al. Factors associated with response to teduglutide in patients with short-bowel syndrome and intestinal failure. Gastroenterology 2018;154:874–85.
59. Lam K, Schwartz L, Batisti J, et al. Single-center experience with the use of teduglutide in adult patients with short bowel syndrome. JPEN J Parenter Enteral Nutr 2018;42:225–30.
60. Schoeler M, Klag T, Wendler J, et al. GLP-2 analog teduglutide significantly reduces need for parenteral nutrition and stool frequency in a real-life setting. Therap Adv Gastroenterol 2018;11. 1756284818793343.
61. Pevny S, Maasberg S, Rieger A, et al. Experience with teduglutide treatment for short bowel syndrome in clinical practice. Clin Nutr 2018;38(4):1745–55.
62. Ukleja A, To C, Alvarez A, et al. Long-term therapy with teduglutide in parenteral support-dependent patients with short bowel syndrome: a case series. JPEN J Parenter Enteral Nutr 2018;42:821–5.
63. Kochar B, Long MD, Shelton E, et al. Safety and Efficacy of Teduglutide (Gattex) in patients with Crohn's disease and need for parenteral support due to short bowel syndrome associated intestinal failure. J Clin Gastroenterol 2017;51: 508–11.
64. Chen KS, Xie J, Tang W, et al. Identifying a subpopulation with higher likelihoods of early response to treatment in a heterogeneous rare disease: a post hoc study of response to teduglutide for short bowel syndrome. Ther Clin Risk Manag 2018; 14:1267–77.
65. Schwartz L. Long-term teduglutide for the treatment of patients with intestinal failure associated with short bowel syndrome. Clin Transl Gastroenterol 2016;7: e142.
66. Fujioka K, Jeejeebhoy K, Pape UF, et al. Patients with short bowel on narcotics during 2 randomized trials have abdominal complaints independent of teduglutide. JPEN J Parenter Enteral Nutr 2017;41:1419–22.
67. Thulesen J, Hartmann B, Hare KJ, et al. Glucagon-like peptide 2 (GLP-2) accelerates the growth of colonic neoplasms in mice. Gut 2004;53:1145–50.
68. Ring LL, Nerup N, Jeppesen PB, et al. Glucagon like peptide-2 and neoplasia; a systematic review. Expert Rev Gastroenterol Hepatol 2018;12:257–64.
69. Ukleja A, Alkhairi B, Bejarano P, et al. De Novo Development of Hamartomatous Duodenal Polyps in a Patient With Short Bowel Syndrome During Teduglutide Therapy: A Case Report. JPEN J Parenter Enteral Nutr 2018;42:658–60.
70. Compher C, Gilroy R, Pertkiewicz M, et al. Maintenance of parenteral nutrition volume reduction, without weight loss, after stopping teduglutide in a subset of patients with short bowel syndrome. JPEN J Parenter Enteral Nutr 2011;35:603–9.
71. Vipperla K, O'Keefe SJ. Targeted therapy of short-bowel syndrome with teduglutide: the new kid on the block. Clin Exp Gastroenterol 2014;7:489–95.
72. Slim GM, Lansing M, Wizzard P, et al. Novel long-acting GLP-2 analogue, FE 203799 (Apraglutide), enhances adaptation and linear intestinal growth in a neonatal piglet model of short bowel syndrome with total resection of the ileum. JPEN J Parenter Enteral Nutr 2019. https://doi.org/10.1002/jpen.1500.
73. Wismann P, Pedersen SL, Hansen G, et al. Novel GLP-1/GLP-2 co-agonists display marked effects on gut volume and improves glycemic control in mice. Physiol Behav 2018;192:72–81.
74. Kirby DF, Corrigan ML, Speerhas RA, et al. Home parenteral nutrition tutorial. JPEN J Parenter Enteral Nutr 2012;36:632–44.
75. Levy E, Frileux P, Sandrucci S, et al. Continuous enteral nutrition during the early adaptive stage of the short bowel syndrome. Br J Surg 1988;75:549–53.

76. Vanderhoof JA, Young RJ. Enteral nutrition in short bowel syndrome. Semin Pediatr Surg 2001;10:65–71.
77. Joly F, Dray X, Corcos O, et al. Tube feeding improves intestinal absorption in short bowel syndrome patients. Gastroenterology 2009;136:824–31.
78. Avitzur Y, Courtney-Martin G. Enteral approaches in malabsorption. Best Pract Res Clin Gastroenterol 2016;30:295–307.
79. Hua Z, Turner JM, Mager DR, et al. Effects of polymeric formula vs elemental formula in neonatal piglets with short bowel syndrome. JPEN J Parenter Enteral Nutr 2014;38:498–506.
80. Buchman AL. Use of percutaneous endoscopic gastrostomy or percutaneous endoscopic jejunostomy in short bowel syndrome. Gastrointest Endosc Clin N Am 2007;17:787–94.

Hepatobiliary Complications of Chronic Intestinal Failure

André Van Gossum, MD, PhD[a],*, Pieter Demetter, MD, PhD[b]

KEYWORDS

- Parenteral nutrition • Home parenteral nutrition • Liver
- Intestinal failure-associated liver disease • Biliary stone • Cholestasis • Steatosis

KEY POINTS

- Intestinal failure-associated liver disease is a multifactorial and complex disorder.
- In young infants, cholestasis is the major component that may rapidly progress to liver failure.
- Diagnosis is based on biochemical, clinical. and histologic alterations; ultra-short gut, lack of enteral nutrition, recurrent sepsis, and parenteral overfeeding are the major risk factors.
- Prevention of harmful factors may strongly decrease the risk for developing intestinal failure-associated liver disease.
- Biliary stone formation in patients on home parenteral nutrition is mostly due to lack of oral/enteral feeding.

INTRODUCTION

Intestinal failure is defined as "the reduction of gut function below the minimum necessary for the absorption of macronutrients and/or water and electrolytes, such that intravenous supplementation is required to maintain health and/or growth."[1] Three subtypes have been described.[2] Type 1 intestinal failure is short term, with a self-limiting requirement for parenteral nutrition (PN), mostly in patients in an intensive care unit. Type 2 is a prolonged acute condition, often in metabolically unstable patients, requiring complex multidisciplinary care and intravenous supplementation over periods of weeks or months. Type 3 intestinal failure is a chronic condition, generally requiring long-term nutritional support in metabolically stable patients. It may be reversible or irreversible. Long-term home PN (HPN) may provoke complications either septic or nonseptic venous access complications or metabolic ones that mainly include liver disorders or bone disease.

Disclosure Statement: The authors have nothing to disclose.
[a] Department of Gastroenterology, Hôpital Erasme/Institut Bordet, Université Libre de Bruxelles, Route de Lennik 808, Brussels B–1070, Belgium; [b] Department of Pathology, Institut Bordet, rue Heger Bordet, 1-1000 Brussels, Belgium
* Corresponding author.
E-mail address: Andre.vangossum@erasme.ulb.ac.be

Gastroenterol Clin N Am 48 (2019) 551–564
https://doi.org/10.1016/j.gtc.2019.08.008

INTESTINAL FAILURE–ASSOCIATED LIVER DISEASE: DEFINITION

Long-term PN has been for long time considered as the sole causative agent for the liver alterations that may occur in patients with IF requiring PN. It used to be named as HPN-related liver disease or HPN-associated liver disease.[3,4] Being multifactorial, it is more appropriate to talk about intestinal failure-associated liver disease (IFALD) in case of use of PN in adult patients with chronic intestinal failure.[5] PN-associated liver disease refers to liver abnormalities that can be observed in infants on PN.

The terminology of PN-associated cholestasis is preferably used in case of cholestasis affecting premature or young infants who are receiving PN.[6] Indeed, cholestasis that may progress to liver failure—in some cases rapidly—is the major feature in this pediatric population. The incidence varies from 20% to 35% of the cases. In infants, PN-associated cholestasis is defined as a concentration of direct bilirubin of more than 2 mg/dL on 2 consecutive measurements (**Box 1**).

There is no standardized definition of IFALD such that the term refers to liver alteration that may occur because of multiple factors that are related to chronic intestinal failure.[7]

The duration and composition of PN may play a role. However, other factors have been identified: episodes of sepsis, lack of enteral nutrition, residual intestinal anatomy, and an ultra-short gut. Moreover, at any other parenchymal liver pathology (eg, viral, autoimmune, nonalcoholic steatohepatitis) or hepatotoxic factors (eg, alcohol, drugs) or biliary obstruction[4,5,8] (**Boxes 2** and **3**).

Most study definitions of IFALD vary and usually rely on biochemical abnormalities rather than histologic characteristics. Liver biopsies have been performed only in a few studies.[9] Study definitions are heterogeneous, including terms such as "abnormal liver function tests," "chronic cholestasis," and "advanced" or "severe liver disease."[10,11]

PREVALENCE OF INTESTINAL FAILURE–ASSOCIATED LIVER DISEASE

Historically, chronic abnormalities in liver function have been reported to occur during HPN in both children and adults, with a wide frequency ranging from 15% to 85% in several series.[3,4,11] In a prospective cohort study of 90 long-term HPN centers in France (1985–1996), 58 patients (65%) developed chronic cholestasis and 37 (42%) developed a severe liver disease after 6 months and 17 months, respectively.[12] Among these patients, 22 showed histologically proven extensive fibrosis (n = 17) or cirrhosis (n = 5) after 27 months (range, 2–148 months). However, it should be noted that these patients were receiving high dose of soy bean-based lipid emulsion.

Box 1
Various terms of liver disorders in pediatric and adult patients on HPN

- HPN-related liver disease
- HPN-associated liver disease
- IFALD[a]
- PN-associated liver disease[b]
- PN-associated cholestasis[c]

[a] To be used in adults.

[b] Currently used in pediatric patients.

[c] Used in pediatric patients with cholestasis.

Box 2
IFALD risk factors in adult patients with HPN

PN

- Energy overfeeding
- Glucose overload >7 mg/kg/min
- Lipid emulsion (LCT) overload
- Soybean LE >1 g/kg/d
- Continuous infusion (24/24 h)
- Contaminants (phytosterols)
- Antioxidant deficiency
- Nutrient deficiency[a] (choline, carnitine, methionine, taurine, essential fatty acid deficiency, etc)

Intestinal failure

- Lack of oral feeding
- Short bowel syndrome (small bowel remnant <50 cm)

Inflammation/infection

- Sepsis (central venous catheter related, etc)
- Small bowel bacterial
- Overgrowth (small intestinal bacterial overgrowth)
- Gut inflammation

Hepatotoxic co-actor

- Chronic alcohol abuse
- Viral infection (C, B)
- Autoimmune
- Hepatotoxic medications

[a] Potential role.

Sasdelli and colleagues[9] recently reported the results of a cross-sectional and retrospective study that included 113 patients in a single center. IFALD was diagnosed by 9 criteria based on liver function rests and liver ultrasound imaging. IFALD diagnoses were categorized as steatosis, cholestasis, or fibrosis. At cross-sectional evaluation, the IFALD prevalence range in each diagnostic category was as follows: cholestasis 5% to 15%, steatosis 17% to 43%, and fibrosis 10% to 20%. At baseline evaluation (initiation of HPN), the IFALD prevalence range was as follows: cholestasis 13% to 40%, steatosis 27% to 90%, and fibrosis 2% to 5%. Notably, IFALD criteria normalized in various porcentages (2%–70%), depending on the diagnostic categories, between baseline and cross-sectional. The authors underlined that IFALD can be present at HPN initiation but may resolve thereafter. The actual prevalence of IFALD is undetermined owing to the lack of a well-defined definition and the changes in the composition of PN during the last decade.

Joly and colleagues[13] reported the results of a multicenter international questionnaire-based retrospective follow-up of 472 patients on HPN. The overall survival probability was 88%, 74%, and 64%, at 1, 3, and 5 years, respectively. By

---

Box 3
Risk factors for developing IFALD in children (premature or newborn infants)

- Prematurity
- Low birth body weight
- Young age at PN commencement
- Frequent episodes of bacterial infections or sepsis
- Long duration of PN
- Fasting or low enteral intake
- Very short gut
- The presence of short bowel syndrome with a stoma
- The presence of gastroschisis or intestinal atresia
- Nutrition
  - High parenteral energy intake
  - Use of soybean-based lipid emulsion >1 g/kg
  - Dextrose infusion >7 mg/kg/min
  - Deficiency of transsulfuration pathway (choline)
  - Toxicity from plant phytosterols
  - Quality and quantity of amino acids

---

the end of the study, 104 patients (23%) died while on HPN, but fewer than 10% of deaths were due to liver disorders.[13]

DIAGNOSIS OF INTESTINAL FAILURE–ASSOCIATED LIVER DISEASE

IFALD should be diagnosed by the presence of abnormal liver function tests and/or evidence of radiologic and/or histologic liver abnormalities occurring in an individual with intestinal failure, in the absence of another parenchymal liver pathology or other hepatotoxic factors or biliary obstruction.[7]

Although liver histology is considered as the gold standard for determining a liver disorder, liver histology is not mandatory for diagnosing IFALD and the decision to perform a liver biopsy should be made on a case-by-case basis. In most cases, a liver biopsy is performed when the patient is considered a candidate for an intestinal transplantation.[7,14]

The presentation of IFALD range from mild cholestasis or steatosis to cirrhosis and decompensated liver disease. In some cases, liver failure may occur without underlying disease and be reversible.[5]

The Paris team defined chronic cholestasis in long-term HPN adult patients as at least a 1.5-fold the upper limit of normal on 2 of 3 liver function measures (γ-glutamyl transferase, alkaline phosphatase, and serum conjugated bilirubin) persistent for at least 6 months.[12] Luman and Shaffer[15] defined IFALD as any biochemical parameter of liver function that was 1.5-fold greater than the reference range when performed at least 6 months after starring HPN.

Imaging techniques including ultrasound examination, computed tomography scan, or MRI cannot certify the diagnosis of IFALD, but can exclude other causes of cholestasis.[4,7,14] Transient elastography (TE) has been proposed as a noninvasive alternative to liver biopsy analysis for assessment of the progression of hepatic fibrosis to cirrhosis.

In a multicenter prospective study, patients receiving long-term HPN (>6 months) who required a liver biopsy for clinical reasons were evaluated by TE (Fibroscan,

Echosens, France).[16] TE values for each patient were compared with the degree of hepatic fibrosis (Brunt classification) and correlated with biochemical and histologic cholestasis. There was no correlation between the values of TE and the stages of histologic fibrosis but TE values were significantly correlated to serum bilirubin level and the severity of histologic cholestasis. Long-term prospective studies starting at initiation of HPN should be performed in adults. Indeed, Hukkinen and colleagues[17] have described that both TE and APRI are promising noninvasive methods for monitoring the development of IFALD in pediatric intestinal failure.

INTESTINAL FAILURE–ASSOCIATED LIVER DISEASE: HISTOLOGIC PATTERNS

It is common to distinguish 2 main categories of hepatic disorders: steatosis and cholestasis.[18,19] This distinction is probably arbitrary regarding the heterogeneity of liver alterations that may be observed in patients with a so-called IFALD. In fact, histologic abnormalities associated with IFALD include steatosis, portal inflammation, portal edema, ductal reaction, ductopenia, and portal and perivenular fibrosis (**Figs. 1–6**). Unlike infants, adults are more likely to demonstrate steatosis and are less susceptible to hepatocellular injury or cholestasis.[4–7,19,20] Moreover, the rate of progression of liver dysfunction in adults varies and does not always correlate with alteration of liver enzymes.

Steatosis seems to be an early complication of PN in adults. Initially, fat accumulation is periportal but with more severe steatosis, the fat distribution is more panlobular or centrilobular. This condition is benign, most of the time asymptomatic, and reversible. Elevation of transaminases is the major biochemical feature.[4–15] The development of steatosis is considered to be due to excess calorie content of PN, especially in the form of carbohydrates. It was quite common at the time of the so-called hyperalimentation. At the histologic level, cholestasis start with a mixed lymphocytic and neutrophilic periportal infiltration, before progression to fibrosis and eventually the development of cirrhosis. Although it is possible, the development of biochemical cholestasis does not progress systematically to fibrosis and/or cirrhosis.[9–20]

PATHOPHYSIOLOGY

The mechanism for developing cholestasis remains unclear and is probably multifactorial (**Figs. 7** and **8**). The liver and intestine play crucial roles in maintaining bile acid

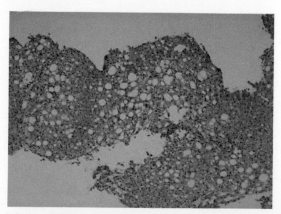

Fig. 1. Diffuse panlobular steatosis (hematoxylin-eosin stain, original magnification ×40).

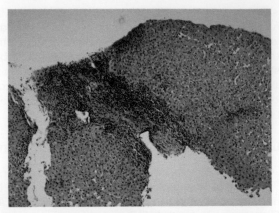

Fig. 2. Portal inflammation (hematoxylin-eosin stain, original magnification ×40).

homeostasis.[21] It has been shown that fibroblast growth factor (FGF) 15 signals from intestine to liver to repress the gene coding cholesterol 7 alpha-hydroxylase, which catalyzes the first and rate-limiting step in the classical bile acid synthetic pathway. FGF 15 expression is stimulated in the small intestine by the nuclear bile acid receptor farnesoid X-activated receptor and repress cholesterol 7 alpha-hydroxylase in liver through a mechanism that involves FGF receptor 4 and the orphan nuclear receptor SHP.[22,23]

Thus, it is known that bile acids activate signal transduction pathways through binding to the specific bile acid receptors TGR5 and farnesoid X-activated receptor. Indirectly, bile acids influence metabolism via modification of the gut microbiota ecosystem. The relation between bile acid metabolism and gut microbiota composition is very complex, and the gut microbiota modulates the bile acid structure, creating a complex bile acid pool consisting of a mixture of differentially structured species; bile acids alter gut microbiota by disturbing bacterial membrane integrity.[24]

In a mouse model, assessing the parenteral-associated cholestasis, El Kasmi and colleagues[25] have observed the role of hepatic macrophages, showing that IL-1 β increased hepatocyte nuclear factor-κB signaling, which interferes with farnesoid X receptor and liver X receptor bonding to respective promoters of canalicular bile and

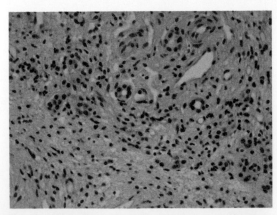

Fig. 3. Ductal reaction (hematoxylin-eosin stain, original magnification ×100).

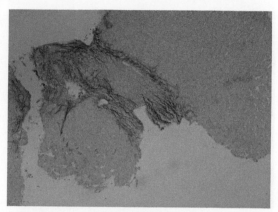

Fig. 4. Portal fibrosis (picrosirius red stain, original magnification ×40).

sterol transporter genes, resulting in transcriptional suppression and subsequent cholestasis. However, in an recent experimental that was performed a novel 90% gut-resected short bowel syndrome model in piglets, Villalona and colleagues[26] noted that, unlike in animals with intact gut, in an animal model of short bowel syndrome there was inadequate chenodeoxycholic acid-induced activation of gut-derived signaling (gut FGF 19 or hepatic farnesoid X-activated receptor, FGF 19, FGF receptor 4) to cause liver improvement. The authors speculated that the activation of the gut liver cross-talk is critically dependent on the presence of adequate gut. They suggested that bile acids therapy may not be as effective for patients with short bowel syndrome.

The factors that may contribute for developing IFALD are numerous.[27] Sepsis seems to be a major factor. It has been especially described in retrospective studies of PN in pediatric patients.[28] It has been postulated that antibiotic therapy might inhibit bacterial translocation and protect liver function in patients with small bowel bacterial overgrowth. Although 2 small studies demonstrated that metronidazole stabilized or improved liver biochemistry in adults receiving short-term PN, there are no strong data for supporting the use of prophylactic use of antibiotics to prevent IFALD in

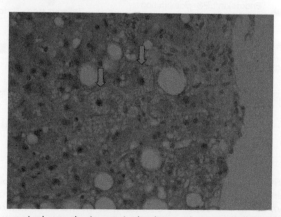

Fig. 5. Mixed macrovesicular and microvesicular (arrows) steatosis (hematoxylin-eosin stain, original magnification ×200).

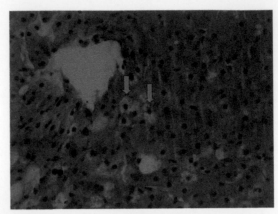

Fig. 6. Microvesicular steatosis (arrows) (hematoxylin-eosin stain, original magnification ×200).

chronic intestinal failure.[14] Several studies demonstrated that a very short gut (<100 cm) was an independent factor for developing chronic cholestasis. The presence of colon in continuity decrease the risk of IFALD. However, this anatomic factor may biased by the need of the requirement in PN.[13–19]

Adaba and colleagues[29] recently published a study aiming to determine the prevalence of chronic cholestasis and whether restoring bowel continuity after a mesenteric infarction decreased the risk of chronic cholestasis. In this study, chronic cholestasis was defined as 2 of bilirubin, alkaline phosphatase, and gamma-glutamyl transferase being 1.5 times the upper limit of normal for more than 6 months. They identified 104 patients (median age, 54 years). Seventy-three patients had restoration of bowel

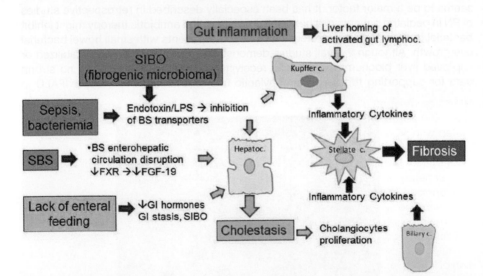

Fig. 7. IFALD: nutrition-related mechanisms. BS, biliary salt; FXR, farnesoid X-activated receptor; GI, gastrointestinal; LPS, lipopolysaccharide; SIBO, small intestinal bacterial overgrowth. (*Data from* Lacaille F, Gupte G, Colomb V, et al. Intestinal-failure associated liver disease: a position paper of the ESPGHAN Working Group of Intestinal Failure and Intestinal Transplantation. J Pediatr Gastroenterol Nutr 2015;60:272–83.)

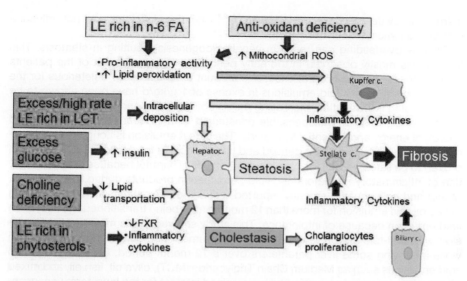

Fig. 8. IFALD: patient-related mechanisms. FA, fatty acids; FXR, farnesoid X-activated receptor; LCT, long chain triglyceride; LE, lipid emulsion; ROS, reactive oxygen species. (*Data from* Lacaille F, Gupte G, Colomb V, et al. Intestinal-failure associated liver disease: a position paper of the ESPGHAN Working Group of Intestinal Failure and Intestinal Transplantation. J Pediatr Gastroenterol Nutr 2015;60:272–83.)

continuity; of these, 25 (34%) had abnormal liver biochemistry, with 15 (21%) having chronic cholestasis. After restoration of bowel continuity, 8 of 15 patients (53%) with chronic cholestasis normalized their liver function within 1 year. Univariate analysis showed restoring bowel continuity ($P = .002$) and cessation of PN ($P = .006$) were associated with a decrease in the prevalence of chronic cholestasis. Multivariate analysis showed that cessation of PN was a significant factor for decreasing chronic cholestasis ($P = .02$).

Cazals-Hatem and colleagues[20] recently reported a series of 32 patients (mean age, 46 years; range, 29–60 years) with irreversible intestinal failure and who underwent a liver biopsy between 2000 and 2013. They underwent liver biopsy 55 months (range, 9–201 months) after beginning HPN. Twenty-six patients (81%) had a short bowel (gut <200 cm). Eighteen patients (56%) had liver fibrosis (4 F2, 10 F3, and 4 F4) associated with steatohepatitis (72%) and/or cholestasis (17%). Factors associated with the occurrence of liver fibrosis included an ultra-short bowel (83% vs 13% at 60 months; $P = .01$), alcohol consumption (73% vs 33% at 60 months; $P<.001$), and diabetes (80% vs 34% at 60 months; $P = .01$). HPN composition, quantity, duration, episodes of sepsis, abandoned bowel segment were not associated with fibrosis. Ultra-short bowel and alcohol consumption independently predicted the development of liver fibrosis on multivariable analysis.

The lack of enteral stimulation has been suspected to play a role in IFALD. However, it is difficult to distinguish the benefit of increasing oral/enteral feeding from the reduction of PN. A cyclic PN modality is preferable and improves the quality of life of patients requiring long-term HPN.[13,14]

The composition of PN itself may contribute to hepatic disorder. Protein and/or essential fatty acid deficiency is associated with steatosis in animal studies. Deficiencies in choline, carnitine, and taurine can result in hepatic steatosis and chronic cholestasis.[30,31] Although some studies show a benefit of supplementation in children, there is no evidence of benefit in adults.[14–32] Carnitine deficiency did not influence IFALD in an international study in adults.[30]

Glucose overfeeding can result in hepatic lipogenesis resulting in steatosis. This finding was mostly observed in the early period of HPN when most of the patients were overfed. The provision of excessive amount of lipid may be deleterious for the liver; soy bean-based lipid emulsions in excess of 1 g/kg/d have been shown to be detrimental to liver function, increasing the risk of morbidity and mortality.[12]

Lipid emulsion is an indispensable constituent of PN because it is a very good source of energy and essential fatty acids. The oldest emulsion is Long Chain Triglyceride (LCT), which is soybean derived and has been used for decades. LCT has been proven to be safe and well tolerated, but is potentially harmful because of the production of inflammatory mediators and lipid peroxidation products during long-term PN. Mundi and colleagues[33] recently reported a series of 17 patients who have used a mixed oil lipid emulsion for more than 12 months after being transitioned from soybean lipid emulsion because of intolerance. This study showed that a mixed oil lipid emulsion was well-tolerated and allowed an improvement in macronutrient composition while improving some liver parameters over a 12-month period. So new generation lipid emulsions such as Medium Chain Triglyceride (MCT), olive oil, fish oil, and mixed oil have been proven to be safe and have gained interest for the long-term use, especially in children.[34–39] However, long-term randomized studies are still needed to confirm this hypothesis and to show an impact not only on biochemical markers, but also on histologic alterations and mortality.

TREATMENT

Treatment of IFALD must start with prevention.[14,30] The European Society for Parenteral and Enteral Nutrition-Home Artificial Nutrition (HAN) chronic intestinal failure group recommend to prevent or manage any episode of sepsis as soon as possible, to attempt preserving small intestinal length and retaining the colon in continuity with the small bowel, to maintain oral and/or enteral nutrition, to avoid PN overfeeding, and to limit the dose of soybean oil-based lipids to less than 1 g/d.[14] There are currently no data to support the role of lipid-free regimens to treat IFALD. Although promising data about the use of pure fish oil emulsion or newer combination lipid emulsions are emerging, more data are required before recommending their use in a routine practice.[14]

As mentioned, any pharmacologic approaches including ursodeoxycholic acid, choline, taurine, or carnitine cannot currently be recommended to treat IFALD in adults with chronic intestinal failure.[30–32]

Impending or overt liver failure is an indication for small bowel/multivisceral transplantation.[40]

The European Society for Parenteral and Enteral Nutrition-HAN-chronic intestinal failure group performed a prospective 5-year study comparing 389 noncandidates and 156 candidates for intestinal transplantation.[41] The primary cause of death on HPN was underlying disease-related in patients with HPN duration less than 2 years, and HPN-related in those on HPN duration for more than 2 years. In transplant candidates, the death hazard ratios were significantly increased in those with desmoids or liver failure. This study confirmed that desmoids and IFALD constitute indications for life-saving intestinal transplantation.

BILIARY-ASSOCIATED COMPLICATIONS OF HOME PARENTERAL NUTRITION

Patients on PN have long been recognized as being at risk for developing cholesterol-based biliary sludge or cholelithiasis.[11] In 2 retrospective studies that included patients with short bowel on HPN, the prevalence of cholelithiasis was 31% and 43%, respectively.[42,43] Several risk factors for developing sludge or cholelithiasis have been identified, including a very short gut, a previous ileocecal valve resection, the duration of HPN, and Crohn's disease as the underlying disease; however, the absence of oral/enteral feeding is most influential.[11,44,45]

Dray and colleagues[46] reported a retrospective study of 153 patients who received HPN for more than 2 months. Of the 119 patients with gallbladder in situ cholelithiasis occurred during HPN in 45 (38%). Biliary complications developed in 8 patients (7%) during follow-up. Therapy consisted of endoscopic sphincterotomy (3 patients) or cholecystectomy (5 patients) with uncomplicated outcomes except for 1 patient; there were no deaths. Although the incidence of developing cholelithiasis in HPN patients is high, the rate of biliary complications is low. This finding is probably due to bile stasis during fasting with a lack of production of cholecystokinin hormone, which is expected to empty the gallbladder.[47] Besides fasting, the administration of lipid emulsion or the use of narcotics could contribute to sludge formation.[48,49]

The use of some drugs such as sincalide (cholecystokinin),[50] intravenous cheno-deoxycholate,[51] or octreotide[52,53] was not really recognized as efficacious for preventing sludge formation. Although it was promoted in the 1980s, prophylactic cholecystectomy is no longer a recommendation.[43] In practice, the major recommendation for preventing the formation of cholelithiasis is to resume as fast as possible oral and/or enteral feeding. The use of narcotics or anticholinergics should be limited as much as possible. Besides these recommendations, treatment for a biliary stone is similar to that in the general population.[14]

SUMMARY

Patients with chronic intestinal failure requiring long-term PN may develop complications, including hepatobiliary disorders. Although there is no standardized definition for IFALD, hepatic disorders are quite frequent in patients on HPN. The prevalence is not well-defined. IFALD is a multifactorial and complex process that includes patient-related variables mainly, ultra-short gut, lack of enteral nutrition, episodes of sepsis, and nutrition-related factors, mainly hyperalimentation and an excess of soybean-based lipid emulsion.

Histologic changes that can be observed in patients with IFALD are numerous. The diagnosis of IFALD is based on clinical, biochemical, and histologic alterations. Prevention of harm is the best treatment. Liver failure is a recognized indication for intestinal multivisceral transplantation. The formation of biliary sludge or stone is common in patients on HPN. A prolonged lack of enteral nutrition is the main factor. Prophylactic cholecystectomy in patients with chronic intestinal failure is not recommended.

REFERENCES

1. Pironi L, Arends J, Baxter J, et al. ESPEN endorsed recommendations. Definition and classification of intestinal failure in adults. Clin Nutr 2015;34:171–80.
2. Pironi L, Konrad D, Brandt C, et al. Clinical classification of adult patients with chronic intestinal failure due to benign disease: an international multicenter cross-sectional survey. Clin Nutr 2018;37:728–38.
3. Quigley EM, Marsh MN, Shaffer JL, et al. Hepatobiliary complications of total parenteral nutrition. Gastroenterology 1993;104:286–301.
4. Bon Djemah V, Colomb V, Corcos O, et al. Home parenteral nutrition-associated liver disease. In: Bozzetti F, Staun M, Van Gossum A, editors. Home parenteral nutrition, 2nd edition. Wallingford, UK:CABI; p. 155–70.

5. Hvas C, Kodjabashia K, Nixon E, et al. Reversal of intestinal failure-associated liver disease (IFALD): emphasis on its multifactorial nature. Frontline Gastroenterol 2016;7:114–7.

6. Vongbhavit K, Underwood M. Predictive value of aspartate aminotransferase to platelet ratio index for parenteral nutrition-associated cholestasis in premature infants with intestinal perforation. JPEN J Parenter Enteral Nutr 2018;42:797–804.

7. Lal S, Pironi L, Wanten G, et al. Clinical approach to the management of Intestinal Failure Associated Liver Disease (IFALD) in adults: a position paper from the Home Artificial Nutrition and Chronic Intestinal Failure Special Interest Group of ESPEN. Clin Nutr 2018;37:1794–7.

8. Canovai E, Ceulemans LJ, Peers G, et al. Cost analysis of chronic intestinal failure. Clin Nutr 2019;38(4):1729–36.

9. Sasdelli AS, Agostini F, Pazzeschi C, et al. Assessment of intestinal failure associated liver disease according to different diagnostic criteria. Clin Nutr 2019;38(3):1198–205.

10. Lindor KD, Fleming CR, Abrams A, et al. Liver function values in adults receiving total parenteral nutrition. JAMA 1979;241:2398–400.

11. Kelly DA. Intestinal failure associated liver disease: what do we know today? Gastroenterology 2006;130(2 suppl 1):S70–7.

12. Cavicchi M, Beau P, Crenn P, et al. Prevalence of liver disease and contributing factors in patients receiving home parenteral nutrition for permanent intestinal failure. Ann Intern Med 2000;132:525–32.

13. Joly F, Baxter J, Staun M, et al. Five-year survival and causes of death in patients on home parenteral nutrition for severe chronic and benign intestinal failure. Clin Nutr 2018;37:1415–22.

14. Pironi L, Arends J, Bozzetti F, et al. ESPEN guidelines on chronic intestinal failure in adults. Clin Nutr 2016;35:247–307.

15. Luman W, Shaffer JL. Prevalence, outcome and associated factors of deranged liver function tests in patients on home parenteral nutrition. Clin Nutr 2002;21:337–43.

16. Van Gossum A, Pironi L, Messing B, et al. Transient elastography (FibroScan) is not correlated with liver fibrosis but with cholestasis in patients with long-term home parenteral nutrition. JPEN J Parenter Enteral Nutr 2015;39:719–24.

17. Hukkinen M, Kivisaari R, Lohi J, et al. Transient elastography and aspartate aminotransferase to platelet ratio predict liver injury in paediatric intestinal failure. Liver Int 2016;36:361–9.

18. Lloyd DAJ, Zabron AA, Gabe SM. Chronic biochemical cholestasis in patients receiving home parenteral nutrition: prevalence and predisposing factors. Aliment Pharmacol Ther 2008;27:552–60.

19. Messing B, Colombel JF, Heresbach D, et al. Chronic cholestasis and macronutrient excess in patients treated with prolonged parenteral nutrition. Nutrition 1992;8:30–6.

20. Cazals-Hatem D, Billiauw L, Rautou PE, et al. Ultrashort bowel is an independent risk factor for liver fibrosis in adults with home parenteral nutrition. Liver Int 2018;38:174–82.

21. Neelis E, de Koning B, Rings E, et al. The gut microbiome in patients with intestinal failure: current evidence and implications for clinical practice. JPEN J Parenter Enteral Nutr 2019;43:194–2005.

22. Inagaki T, choi M, Moschetta A, et al. Fibroblast growth factor 15 functions as an enterohepatic signal to regulate bile acid homeostasis. Cell Metab 2005;2:217–25.

23. Makishima M, Okamoto A, Repa JJ, et al. Identification of a nuclear receptor for bile acids. Science 1999;284:1362–5.

24. Boesjes M, Brufau G. Metabolic effects of bile acids in the gut in health and disease. Curr Med Chem 2014;21:2822–9.

25. El Kasmi K, Vue P, Anderson A, et al. Macrophage-derived IL-1β-kB signaling mediates parenteral nutrition-associated cholestasis. Nat Commun 2018;9:1393.

26. Villalona G, Price A, Blomenkamp K, et al. No gut no gain! Enteral bile acid treatment preserves gut growth but not parenteral nutrition-associated liver injury in a novel extensive short bowel animal model. JPEN J Parenter Enteral Nutr 2018;42: 1238–51.

27. Rochling FA, Catron HA. Intestinal failure-associated liver disease: causes, manifestations and therapies. Curr Opin Gastroenterol 2019;35(2):126–33.

28. Clare A, Teubner A, Shaffer JL. What information should lead to a suspicion of catheter sepsis in HPN? Clin Nutr 2008;27:552–6.

29. Adaba F, Uppara M, Iqbal F, et al. Chronic cholestasis in patients on parenteral nutrition: the influence of restoring bowel continuity after mesenteric infarction. Eur J Clin Nutr 2016;70:189–93.

30. Bowyer BA, Miles JM, Haymond MW, et al. L-Carnitine therapy in home parenteral nutrition patients with abnormal liver tests and low plasma carnitine concentrations. Gastroenterology 1988;94:434–8.

31. Buchman AL, Ament ME, Sohel M, et al. Choline deficiency causes reversible hepatic abnormalities in patients receiving parenteral nutrition: proof of a human choline requirement: a placebo controlled trial. JPEN J Parenter Enteral Nutr 2001;25:260–8.

32. Buchman AL, Dubin M, Jenden D, et al. Lecithin increases plasma free choline and decreases hepatic steatosis in long-term total parenteral nutrition patients. Gastroenterology 1992;102(4 Pt 1):1363–70.

33. Mundi MS, Kuchkuntla AR, Salonen BR, et al. Long-term use of mixed-oil lipid emulsion in soybean oil-intolerant home parenteral nutrition patients. JPEN J Parenter Enteral Nutr 2019. [Epub ahead of print].

34. Pironi L, Colecchia A, Guidetti M, et al. Fish oil-based emulsion for the treatment of parenteral nutrition associated liver disease in an adult patient. e-SPEN 2010;5: e243–6.

35. Burns DL, Gill BM. Reversal of parenteral nutrition-associated liver disease with a fish oil-based lipid emulsion (Omegaven) in an adult dependent on home parenteral nutrition. JPEN J Parenter Enteral Nutr 2013;37:274–80.

36. Venecourt-Jackson E, Hill SJ, Walmsley RS. Successful treatment of parenteral nutrition-associated liver disease in an adult by use of a fish oil-based lipid source. Nutrition 2013;29:356–8.

37. Xu Z, Li Y, Wang J, et al. Effect of omega-3 polyunsaturated fatty acids to reverse biopsy-proven parenteral nutrition-associated liver disease in adults. Clin Nutr 2012;31:217–23.

38. Klek S, Szczepanek K, Scislo L, et al. Intravenous lipid emulsions and liver function in adult chronic intestinal failure patients: results from a randomized clinical trial. Nutrition 2018;55-56:45–50.

39. Wang C, Venick RS, Shew SB, et al. Long-term outcomes in children with intestinal failure-associated liver disease treated with 6 months of intravenous fish oil followed by resumption of intravenous soybean oil. JPEN J Parenter Enteral Nutr 2019;43(6):708–16.

40. Pironi L, Goulet O, Buchman A, et al. Outcome on home parenteral nutrition for benign intestinal failure: a review of the literature and benchmarking with the European prospective survey of ESPEN. Clin Nutr 2012;31:831–45.

41. Pironi L, Joly F, Forbes A, et al. Long-term follow-up of patients on home parenteral nutrition in Europe: implications for intestinal transplantation. Gut 2011;60: 17–25.

42. Nightingale JM, Lennard-Jones JE, Gertner D, et al. Colonic preservation reduces need for parenteral therapy, increases incidence of renal stones, but does not change high prevalence of gallstones in patients with a short bowel. Gut 1992;33:1493–7.

43. Thompson JS. The role of prophylactic cholecystectomy in the short-bowel syndrome. Arch Surg 1996;131(5):556–9.

44. Messing B, Bories C, Kunstlinger F, et al. Does total parenteral nutrition induce gallbladder sludge formation and lithiasis? Gastroenterology 1983;84:1012–9.

45. Lapidus A, Einarsson C. Bile composition in patients with ileal resection due to Crohn's disease. Inflamm Bowel Dis 1998;4:89–94.

46. Dray X, Joly F, Reijasse D, et al. Incidence, risk factors, and complications of cholelithiasis in patients with home parenteral nutrition. J Am Coll Surg 2007; 204:13–21.

47. Dawes L, Laut H, Woodruff M. Decreased bile acid synthesis with total parenteral nutrition. Am J Surg 2007;194:623–7.

48. Rubin M, Haldern Z, Charach G, et al. Effect of lipid infusion on lipid composition and lithogenicity in patients without cholesterol gallstones. Gut 1992;33:1400–3.

49. Manji N, Bistrian B, Mascioli E, et al. Gallstone disease in patients with severe short bowel syndrome dependent on parenteral nutrition. JPEN J Parenter Enteral Nutr 1989;13:461–4.

50. Prescott WA, Btaiche I. Sincalide in patients with parenteral nutrition associated gallbladder disease. Ann Pharmacother 2004;38:1942–5.

51. Broughton G, Fitzgibbons RJ, Geiss R, et al. IV chenodeoxycholate prevents calcium bilirubinate gallstones during total parenteral nutrition in the prairie dog. JPEN J Parenter Enteral Nutr 1996;20:187–93.

52. Baudet S, Medina C, Vilaseca J, et al. Effect of short-term octreotide therapy and total parenteral nutrition on the development of biliary sludge and lithiasis. Hepatogastroenterology 2002;49:609–12.

53. Pironi L, Sasdelli A. Intestinal failure-associated liver disease. Clin Liver Dis 2019; 23:279–91.

Nontransplant Surgery for Intestinal Failure

Riccardo Colletta, MD, PhD[a,b], Antonino Morabito, MD, FRCS[a,b,c],
Kishore Iyer, MBBS, FRCS (Eng)[d],*

KEYWORDS

- Short bowel syndrome • Adaptation • Dilatation • Autologous reconstruction
- Lengthening

KEY POINTS

- Insufficient absorptive mucosal surface is the fundamental problem in the short bowel state.
- Intestinal adaptation has been well studied, and it is well recognized that it may lead to dilatation of the bowel with increased thickness of the bowel wall, resulting from both mucosal hypertrophy and hyperplasia.
- Autologous reconstructive surgery exploits bowel dilatation in short bowel syndrome and maximizes the absorptive potential of the available mucosal surface.

INTRODUCTION

Bowel resection may lead to loss of absorptive surface area and decreased intestinal transit time. The consequence is often decreased contact of the nutrients with the enteric mucosa and malabsorption. Although previously fatal, long-term survival in patients with intestinal failure (IF) is now expected with the widespread use of parenteral nutrition (PN), introduced by Wilmore and Dudrick,[1] about half a century ago. Over the last few years, considerable advances have been achieved in the medical and surgical management of short bowel syndrome (SBS),[2,3] and nontransplant surgery continues to occupy a key role in the management of these complex patients.

Autologous gastrointestinal reconstructive (AGIR) procedures are often more fine art, as the surgeon tailors the patient's remaining bowel to restore adequate physiology often by improving bowel length. Consequently, effective surgical management

Disclosures: None.
[a] Department of Paediatric Surgery, Center for Intestinal Reconstruction and Rehabilitation, Meyer Children's Hospital, Viale Gaetanao Pieraccini. 24, Florence 50139, Italy; [b] School of Environment and Life Science, University of Salford, Salford, UK; [c] Department of NeuroFarBa, University of Florence, Florence, Italy; [d] Intestinal Rehabilitation & Transplant Program, Icahn School of Medicine at Mount Sinai, Mount Sinai Hospital, One Gustave Levy Place, Box 1104, New York, NY 10029, USA
* Corresponding author.
E-mail address: kishore.iyer@mountsinai.org

of IF requires an accurate understanding of disease origin, remnant bowel length, and other residual anatomic characteristics, such as presence of stomas, blind loops, or colonic remnant.

The initial goal of management in patients with intestinal failure is to wean PN and minimize PN-associated comorbidities. Patient selection in AGIR is essential for good outcomes. To obtain the best possible result from nontransplant surgery, a multidisciplinary approach in reviewing patient's history, including prior surgical notes, review of previous radiological examination, direct conversation with previous surgeons when possible, study of PN formula to reduce liver complications, current progress with PN-weaning, and provision of adequate psychosocial support, is advisable. Such multidisciplinary management, as reviewed by Matarese and colleagues,[4] allows for optimal planning in terms of deployment of different treatment options, evaluation of therapeutic success, and determination of timing for escalated intervention, whether it be surgery or even intestinal transplantation.

The modern era of nontransplant surgery started when Adrian Bianchi described the longitudinal intestinal lengthening and tapering (LILT) procedure in 1982 (see later discussion). At the time, this procedure was developed to prevent the baleful outcome of patients suffering from SBS or IF when long-term PN almost inevitably led to liver disease. In that scenario the only viable option for these patients was intestinal transplant at a time when transplant outcomes were poor. It is of interest to note that the LILT procedure was developed primarily to decrease intestinal stasis and treat small intestinal bacterial overgrowth in patients with dilated bowel, rather than as a means to achieve enteral autonomy. As it happens, the ability to wean patients off PN following AGIR surgery was initially a by-product of surgical treatment of bacterial overgrowth, albeit a very important one.

Surgical management should commence with prevention of SBS and preservation of all possible small bowel in the vulnerable patient. This strategy includes early recognition of high-risk situations for loss of critical bowel lengths and using conservative strategies to avoid preventable bowel loss, thereby potentially improving outcomes. This strategy is important for every pediatric surgeon dealing with intestinal catastrophic events such as necrotizing enterocolitis (NEC) or volvulus due to intestinal malrotation during the neonatal period. These 2 conditions are the main cause of extensive surgical resection but fortunately changes in clinical practice, and improvements in neonatal care, such as the early recognition and medical treatment of NEC, can improve bowel salvage in difficult cases. Furthermore, children with this complex condition have improved survival rates due to a better understanding of PN administration including in the home setting (home parenteral nutrition). Different lipid formulations for PN have been developed and combined with improved understanding of the consequences of administering too much liquid, have reduced dramatically the frequency of intestinal failure–associated liver disease (IFALD). Hepato-sparing PN using lipid restriction (maximum of 1 g/kg/d of intralipid or 2 g/kg/d of SMOF) can be considered the first step in the multidisciplinary management before performing nontransplant surgery. Furthermore, aggressive oral/enteral feeding is strongly recommended to facilitate bowel absorptive function and to improve the possibility of weaning from PN because food aversion has been shown to be one important cause of permanence with a life in total parenteral nutrition (TPN).

BOWEL DILATATION IN SHORT BOWEL SYNDROME

Dilatation of part of the remnant small bowel is a frequent finding in SBS. The exact cause of dilatation is unknown—a teleologic view would suggest that dilatation is part of the process of intestinal adaptation. Personal experience suggests that although this may be true, dilatation is often also seen in watershed areas of the small bowel with marginal blood supply. Whatever the reason, the suspicion that dilated bowel is poorly peristaltic and militates against progress to enteral autonomy has been elegantly studied by Pakarinen's group from Helsinki.[5,6] In a study of 60 eligible children with SBS-IF, Hukkinen and colleagues[5] showed that patients with spontaneous symptomatic dilatation unable to wean off PN underwent intestinal tapering surgery at a median age of 1.04 years (0.70–3.27). SBS children with short remaining small bowel length, missing ileocecal valve, and small bowel atresia as the underlying diagnosis were more likely to require tapering surgery. Of operated patients, 75% of children eventually achieved enteral autonomy from PN similar to non-operated children.[5] In a related study of 61 children, the same group showed that small bowel diameter could be consistently expressed as a ratio to the fifth lumbar vertebra.[6] Weaning off PN was 14-fold more likely with small bowel diameter ratio less than 2.0 compared with greater than 3.0- and 5.4-fold more likely when maximal small bowel diameter was less than 20 mm compared with greater than 30 mm. After adjustment for age, remaining small bowel length and the presence of ileocecal valve, both estimates of maximal small bowel diameter, remained significant independent predictors for weaning off PN. Importantly, when all measurements were included, the cumulative survival was worse if small bowel diameter ratio exceeded 2.0.[6]

NONTRANSPLANT SURGICAL MANAGEMENT PHILOSOPHY

Surgical options in patients with SBS or IF falls into 1 of 3 groups: (1) procedures to improve transit time in the absence of dilatation, (2) procedures to correct or improve intestinal dilatation, and (3) procedures to cause bowel dilatation, in the hope of future surgical exploitation.

The indications for nontransplant surgery for a patient with IF should possibly be considered within the first year of life to successfully progress with weaning from PN. During this period the presence of life-threatening complications such as PN-related liver disease or IFALD, recurrent central line sepsis, and loss of vascular access need to be prevented. Furthermore, nontransplant surgery should not be considered only as a rescue procedure but rather as an integral part of a structured plan toward enteral autonomy, formulated from a multidisciplinary team when the child is first registered with the intestinal failure center. Early surgery should be preventative and directed at preserving all possible bowel.

It is important to emphasize that in this article the authors have chosen not to discuss routine general surgical procedures that in their view fall under the umbrella of good, common sense–driven surgical principles that can be of tremendous value in the care of the patient with SBS. Thus, correction of underlying pathology such as blind loops or enterocutaneous or enteroenteric fistulas is valuable in the patient with SBS, as also recruitment of any distal bowel by early take-down or even avoidance of stomas, but are not discussed further in this article.

Procedures to Improve Intestinal Transit Time in the Absence of Dilatation

Surgical attempts at improving mucosal absorption have been varied and imaginative. Some, such as "recirculating loops" and "pouches," have not proved beneficial. Others, including bowel pacing, neomucosal growth, mucosal stem cell regeneration, and tissue-engineered intestine[7] may yet develop to clinical application.

Reversed (antiperistaltic) segment

In patients with rapid transit time due to extensive bowel resection, in the absence of meaningful bowel dilation, creation of a reverse (antiperistaltic) segment can be a useful option. Reversal of single or multiple segments of small bowel acting antiperistaltically counteracts the tendency to rapid loss of fluid, electrolyte, and nutrient by delaying passage sufficiently for increased absorption. Most reports indicated a definite delay in transit with a beneficial increase in absorption.[8–10] Unfortunately, the length of the reversed segment seems to be critical, such that the procedure may be ineffective or alternatively pathologically obstructive. The length of the segment to reverse is recommended to be between 10 and 15 cm in the adult population and more than 3 cm for the children. Long-term results of segmental reversal of the small bowel were reported from Paris in a cohort of 38 adult patients with "permanent" PN dependence. At a median follow-up of close to 5 years, 45% of patients were weaned off PN. In the remaining patients, PN dependency had been decreased from 7 ± 1 to 4 ± 1 days per week, with an overall survival rate of 84%.[11]

Colonic interposition—isoperistaltic or antiperistaltic

The interposition of a segment of colon between small bowel remnants has been shown to be effective in slowing the rapid intestinal transit that usually occurs in SBS. Colonic interposition was introduced by Hutcher and Salzberg[12] (1973) because the colon has reduced motility compared with small bowel and because of its ability to absorb fluid and electrolytes. Glick and colleagues[13] (1984) published a series of 6 children who had undergone 8 to 15-cm isoperistaltic prejejunal colon placement. Bowel length varied between 21 and 63 cm, and the indications for surgery were enteral intolerance at 5 to 9 months and PN-related complications.

Transposition of the colon does not involve the sacrifice of valuable bowel. It is straightforward and reversible and may tilt the balance favorably for those with sufficient absorptive mucosa but rapid transit.

Interestingly, colonic interposition has also been shown to exhibit adaptive changes that reflect the morphologic and functional features of the small intestine in animal models of SBS.[14,15] The adaptive change of the colon epithelium was also reported in human, where a biopsy specimen revealed that the mucosa of the interposed colon adjacent to the ileum showed hypertrophy and hyperplasia of the crypt glands and cells resembling Paneth cells, which are usually seen in the small intestine.[16] This procedure can be potentially useful either in isolation or as part of a combined bowel nontransplant procedure.

Procedures to Correct Intestinal Dilatation

Longitudinal intestinal lengthening and tapering procedure

LILT was first described in 1980[17] by Adrian Bianchi and then used successfully in the first patient in 1981.[18] The technique involves dividing the longest segment of dilated bowel along the antimesenteric border, with extra care to ensure the highest numbers of blood vessels are preserved. The avascular plane at the mesenteric border of the bowel is then developed taking care to avoid any injury to the mesenteric blood supply. The bowel is then divided into 2 vascularized hemisegments along the mesenteric border. The 2 hemisegments are than tubularized to form hemiloops and anastomosed to each other in an isoperistaltic fashion. Bowel continuity is reestablished with a wide oblique hemiloop anastomosis in the original "lazy S" or the Aigrain spiral.[19] Bowel function usually resumes between 3 and 5 days.[20–22] Recent data show that survival rates with LILT vary between 30% and 100%. Of survivors, post-LILT, 28% to 100% were weaned off PN.[23] The wide range of the results using LILT procedures suggests that surgical experience in performing this technique and the involvement of an experienced multidisciplinary intestinal rehabilitation program may play an important role in ultimate success.

Serial transverse enteroplasty

Serial transverse enteroplasty (STEP), first proposed by Kim and colleagues[24] in 2003, is a procedure that involves a stapler being applied across dilated bowel in an alternating fashion, such that it leaves the bowel in the shape of a zig-zag, leaving a more normalized luminal diameter.[25] The creation of the zig-zag requires a mesenteric defect at each staple line but otherwise does not interfere with the mesenteric blood supply of the bowel. The stapler is placed at 90° and 270°, with 0° being the mesenteric border, and incisions are made in the bowel, leaving the bowel approximately 2 cm in diameter.[26]

The main advantage of this procedure is that STEP lengthens and tailors the bowel, without interfering with the mesenteric blood supply. It is also conceptually relatively simple, and because of the natural redilation of bowel that occurs in many cases, some investigators believe that STEP can be used safely after a dilatation following prior LILT.[27] Multiple STEP procedures can be performed on the same patient after the process of adaptation and dilation has occurred.[28] The bowel is remarkably lengthened during the STEP procedure, with one study on animals showing an average increase of 64%.[26] Barrett and colleagues[29] suggest a need for caution in using multiple STEP procedures, with re-STEPs failing to result in significant PN weaning, and no re-STEP patients achieving enteral autonomy during follow-up. The main reported complications post-STEP are intestinal obstruction, interloop fistulae, and bleeding from the suture line.[27] The occurrence of these complications in a significant percentage of patients reiterates the fact that patients with SBS and IF are medically complex; no single operation represents a panacea, with patient selection for these procedures remaining an important determinant of good outcomes. Questions remain about the physiologic implications of the STEP procedure, as there is a change in orientation of the muscle fibers in the lengthened segment. It is still not clear whether peristalsis is restored in the STEP segment, or the intestine becomes passive, and whether this procedure has any direct impact on the function of the intestine.

Spiral intestinal lengthening and tapering

The newest of the "lengthening" procedures was established on the bench[30] and tested in modeled Vietnamese pigs in 2011.[31] In the original experiment, the animals were kept on water for 24 hours, then given liquid food for 48 to 72 hours postoperatively. Of the 6 pigs that underwent this procedure, 4 had an uneventful postoperative course. Autopsies showed that bowel obstruction did develop in 2 pigs. In both autopsies, the lumen was shown to have narrowed by 70% to a diameter under 1.5 cm. Statistical analysis of the results showed no significant difference in length and width measured immediately after spiral intestinal lengthening and tapering (SILT) and that measured 5 weeks later. All lengthened segments showed peristalsis immediately after the procedure and at terminal laparotomy 5 weeks after or at autopsy.

The procedure involves drawing spiral incision lines at 45 to 60° angles on the bowel. The mesentery is then incised perpendicularly to the marked points. The incisions are now made on the bowel, and the bowel is then stretched longitudinally over an intraluminal catheter to a larger tube of narrower diameter. Finally, the mesenteric defects are narrowed to prevent intraabdominal herniation.

The first SILT procedure for a patient with SBS was performed in Manchester in 2012 with good results. The patient was weaned off TPN after 6 months.[32] A 3-year-old patient born at 24 weeks gestation was deemed suitable for the SILT procedure. After natural intestinal adaptation aided by PN, gastrostomy feeding, structured controlled bowel expansion, and continuous extracorporeal stool recycling (see later discussion), she underwent SILT. Before SILT, the length of the jejunum was increased from 15 cm to 22 cm using controlled tissue expansion, a technique that allows controlled dilation of segments of intestine.[33] Using SILT, the Manchester group extended the 11 cm of distended bowel to 20 cm. Five days after SILT, patient was started on oral and gastrostomy feeding, and there were no surgical complications. She was weaned off PN, with good liver function 6 months after the procedure.

Alberti and colleagues[33] reported the second clinical case of SILT in 2014 where this procedure was performed in a patient with 9 cm of jejunum after a period of controlled bowel expansion. So far, the biggest experience in SILT cases with a median follow-up longer than 24 months was reported in 2018.[34] SILT was applied in 5 consecutive cases of patients with a median age of 8.3 months at procedure. SILT allowed a median increase in length of 56% (10–15 cm; $P<.03$) and tailoring of the dilated segment, providing a reduction in diameter of 50% (4.3–2.1 cm; $P<.01$). During the follow-up period, all patients were gradually weaned off TPN and after 6 months the need of TPN support was reduced from a median of 7 to 4 nights per week. SILT was used not only as a primary AGIR surgery option but also as a combined procedure with STEP.

Procedures to Increase Bowel Dilatation

Controlled tissue expansion

Bowel dilatation can occur either spontaneously during the intestinal adaptation phase or can be triggered by formation of tube stomas. Controlled tissue expansion (CTE) is a surgical approach aiming to dilate remaining bowel in a patient suffering from SBS, with a view to further surgical exploitation by lengthening as mentioned earlier. Bowel expansion is particularly applicable to the child with a nondilated bowel, who may then also benefit from subsequent lengthening procedures.

Creation of nipple valves to cause partial obstruction and consequent dilatation, from autologous tissue rather than prosthetic materials may be better tolerated, but requires the sacrifice of a significant segment of small bowel. Such valves also have the inherent disadvantage of a predetermined fixed degree of bowel obstruction, which may be either ineffective or too tight, and does not allow for dynamic variation toward maximal efficiency.[35]

Bianchi introduced the concept of CTE modifying the nipple valve idea of Georgeson, and the first report was published in 2011.[35]

CTE allows controlled expansion of the bowel as the occlusion of the bowel lumen is monitored and controlled from outside the intestinal lumen, minimizing the risk of bacterial overgrowth and translocation.

Collected proximal jejunal content is recycled down a distal tube colostomy at a slow and steady rate to stimulate mucosal absorption and adaptation also in the distal bowel. Occlusion of the proximal tube jejunostomy for variable periods induces controlled bowel expansion.

This model also allows for direct access to the jejunum for "housekeeping," that is, bacterial cultures, loop washouts, endoscopy, and biopsy. Thus, surgery is minimal, and no bowel is lost or sacrificed. Controlled expansion-recycle can be maintained for several months until sufficient dilatation has been achieved and the child is generally fit for lengthening procedures. Discomfort and pain are minimal as the clamping can be stopped at any time. CTE typically allows bowel dilatation in 20 to 24 weeks. Bowel expansion has the added advantage of inducing mucosal growth, thereby creating new mucosal surface area for absorption.[36]

RESULTS

The first comparison of the 2 main intestinal lengthening procedures (LILT and STEP) was performed in 2007 by Sudan and colleagues[37] from Omaha reporting on a 24-year cumulative experience. Survival, total TPN weaning, and complications were analyzed.[37] Sixty-four patients underwent 43 LILT and 34 STEP procedures but no clear information about bowel dilatation and condition of mesentery were provided. Interestingly, both the procedures showed a survival rate greater than 80% (Bianchi 88%, STEP 95%) with median follow-up of 3.8 years. Both lengthening procedures were associated with an increase in the enteral caloric intake—for pediatric patients increasing from 15 kcal/kg before lengthening to 85 kcal/kg at 1 year after lengthening. Of note, complications occurred in 10% of patients, and intestinal transplantation as salvage therapy was required in 14% of patients at a median of 2.9 years after lengthening. Miyasaka and colleagues[38] reporting from Ann Arbor, Michigan reported on 14 lengthening procedures over a 15-year period. Despite overall good survival rates of 86% for LILT patients and 89% for STEP patients, they reported a high rate of complications (93%) following lengthening and redilatation of the bowel in more than half the patients.[38]

In 2013, a systematic review of these 2 lengthening procedures was performed analyzing 403 patients (276 Bianchi procedures and 127 STEP operation) reported in the literature.[23] Overall survival, especially in the last 15 years was excellent after lengthening procedures. The percentage of patients weaned from TPN was significantly higher in the Bianchi group than in the STEP group, with a higher rate of patients receiving intestinal transplant as salvage. We could speculate that the shorter length of follow-up for STEP patients may have an impact on these results. Complication rates were significantly higher in STEP patients than in LILT patients.[23]

Both LILT and STEP seems to be acceptable procedures with acceptable survival and nutritional outcomes for nontransplant surgical management of SBS in children. Larger studies are needed to further guide accurate selection of eligible patients. A study based on the International STEP Data Registry showed that overall mortality post-STEP was 11%.[39] Pre-STEP risk factors for progressing to transplantation or death were higher direct bilirubin level and shorter bowel length. Among patients who underwent STEP for SBS, 47% attained full enteral nutrition post-STEP. Patients with longer pre-STEP bowel length were significantly more likely to achieve enteral autonomy.[39]

DISCUSSION

Insufficient absorptive mucosal surface is the fundamental problem in the short bowel state. Intestinal adaptation has been well studied, and it is well recognized that it may lead to dilatation of the bowel with increased thickness of the bowel wall, resulting from both mucosal hypertrophy and hyperplasia. Autologous reconstructive surgery exploits bowel dilatation in SBS and maximizes the absorptive potential of the available mucosal surface. Indeed, AGIR may be better viewed as optimizing bowel diameter rather than focusing on length, thus allowing better prograde peristalsis and improved contact between luminal nutrients and mucosa, ultimately enhancing absorption.

A few autologous bowel reconstructive procedures have been described through the years. It is essential to understand that each procedure has its own indication and clinical application, as one size does not fit all. The duty of the bowel reconstructive surgeon is to use the available surgical procedures to meet the individual needs of the patient, with the final goal of nutritional autonomy from PN.

Data from the literature report better outcomes for AGIR in dedicated intestinal rehabilitation centers. Although this may reflect greater surgical expertise in a niche area, it may equally reflect better patient selection as well as the value of an expert multidisciplinary team providing holistic care to the challenging patient with SBS.

In this field, we have now moved toward an individualized medical and surgical approach because each patient has unique needs. The surgical care of the patient with SBS requires a high level of expertise and experience in this field, but it is the key to maintain and indeed optimize outcomes for this otherwise life-threatening condition. With greater understanding of the pathophysiology of IF and the ability to minimize the life-threatening complications of PN, there is ever greater opportunity for the intestinal rehabilitation surgeon to use different surgical techniques to provide the right operation for the right patient at the right time. At the same time, intestinal transplant outcomes steadily improve, with 1-year survival from the experienced centers exceeding 90% for patients, and 5-year survival approaching 70% to 75% with most of the survivors being off PN. Under the circumstances, the intestinal rehabilitation surgeon using nontransplant procedures has even greater responsibility to avoid futile or misguided operations in order to not miss often limited windows of opportunity for successful intestinal transplant, in the patient who is failing conservative medical and surgical care.

REFERENCES

1. Wilmore DW, Dudrick SJ. Growth and development of an infant receiving all nutrients exclusively by vein. JAMA 1968;203(10):860–4.

2. Merras-Salmio L, Mutanen A, Ylinen E, et al. Pediatric intestinal failure: the key outcomes for the first 100 patients treated in a national tertiary referral center during 1984-2017. JPEN J Parenter Enteral Nutr 2018;42(8):1304–13.

3. Brown SK, Davies N, Smyth E, et al. Intestinal failure: the evolving demographic and patient outcomes on home parenteral nutrition. Acta Paediatr 2018;107(12): 2207–11.

4. Matarese LE, Jeppesen PB, O'Keefe SJ. Short bowel syndrome in adults: the need for an interdisciplinary approach and coordinated care. JPEN J Parenter Enteral Nutr 2014;38(1 Suppl):60S–4S.

5. Hukkinen M, Kivisari R, Kolvusalo A, et al. Risk factors and outcomes of tapering surgery for small intestinal dilatation in pediatric short bowel syndrome. J Pediatr Surg 2017;52:1121–7.

6. Hukkinen M, Kivisaari R, Merras-Salmio L, et al. Small bowel dilatation predicts prolonged parenteral nutrition and decreased survival in pediatric short bowel syndrome. Ann Surg 2017;266(2):369–75.

7. Kaihara S, Kim SS, Kim BS, et al. Long-term follow-up of tissue-engineered intestine after anastomosis to native small bowel. Transplantation 2000;69(9):1927–32.

8. Thompson JS, Rikkers LF. Surgical alternatives for the short bowel syndrome. Am J Gastroenterol 1987;82(2):97–106.

9. Pigot F, Messing B, Chaussade S, et al. Severe short bowel syndrome with a surgically reversed small bowel segment. Dig Dis Sci 1990;35(1):137–44.

10. Panis Y, Messing B, Rivet P, et al. Segmental reversal of the small bowel as an alternative to intestinal transplantation in patients with short bowel syndrome. Ann Surg 1997;225(4):401–7.
11. Beyer-berjot L, Joly F, Maggiori L, et al. Segmental reversal of the small bowel can end permanent nutrition depndency: an experience of 38 adults with short bowel syndrome. Ann Surg 2012;256(5):739–44 [discussion: 744–5].
12. Hutcher NE, Salzberg AM. Pre-ileal transposition of colon to prevent the development of short bowel syndrome in puppies with 90 percent small intestinal resection. Surgery 1971;70(2):189–97.
13. Glick PL, de Lorimier AA, Adzick NS, et al. Colon interposition: an adjuvant operation for short-gut syndrome. J Pediatr Surg 1984;19(6):719–25.
14. Sidhu GS, Narasimharao KL, Rani VU, et al. Morphological and functional changes in the gut after massive small bowel resection and colon interposition in rhesus monkeys. Digestion 1984;29(1):47–54.
15. King DR, Anvari M, Jamieson GG, et al. Does the colon adopt small bowel features in a small bowel environment? Aust N Z J Surg 1996;66(8):543–6.
16. Kono K, Sekikawa T, Iizuka H, et al. Interposed colon between remnants of the small intestine exhibits small bowel features in a patient with short bowel syndrome. Dig Surg 2001;18(3):237–41.
17. Bianchi A. Intestinal loop lengthening–a technique for increasing small intestinal length. J Pediatr Surg 1980;15(2):145–51.
18. Boeckman CR, Traylor R. Bowel lengthening for short gut syndrome. J Pediatr Surg 1981;16(6):996–7.
19. Aigrain Y, Cornet D, Cezard JP, et al. Longitudinal division of small intestine: a surgical possibility for children with the very short bowel syndrome. Z Kinderchir 1985;40(4):233–6.
20. Khalil BA, Ba'ath ME, Aziz A, et al. Intestinal rehabilitation and bowel reconstructive surgery: improved outcomes in children with short bowel syndrome. J Pediatr Gastroenterol Nutr 2012;54(4):505–9.
21. Ba'ath ME, Almond S, King B, et al. Short bowel syndrome: a practical pathway leading to successful enteral autonomy. World J Surg 2012;36(5):1044–8.
22. Pakarinen MP. Autologous intestinal reconstruction surgery as part of comprehensive management of intestinal failure. Pediatr Surg Int 2015;31(5):453–64.
23. King B, Carlson G, Khalil BA, et al. Intestinal bowel lengthening in children with short bowel syndrome: systematic review of the Bianchi and STEP procedures. World J Surg 2013;37(3):694–704.
24. Kim HB, Lee PW, Garza J, et al. Serial transverse enteroplasty for short bowel syndrome: a case report. J Pediatr Surg 2003;38(6):881–5.
25. Ching YA, Gura K, Modi B, et al. Pediatric intestinal failure: nutrition, pharmacologic, and surgical approaches. Nutr Clin Pract 2007;22(6):653–63.
26. Kim HB, Fauza D, Garza J, et al. Serial transverse enteroplasty (STEP): a novel bowel lengthening procedure. J Pediatr Surg 2003;38(3):425–0.
27. Modi BP, Javid PJ, Jaksic T, et al. First report of the international serial transverse enteroplasty data registry: indications, efficacy, and complications. J Am Coll Surg 2007;204(3):365–71.
28. Piper H, Modi BP, Kim HB, et al. The second STEP: the feasibility of repeat serial transverse enteroplasty. J Pediatr Surg 2006;41(12):1951–6.
29. Barrett M, Demehri FR, Ives GC, et al. Taking a STEP back: Assessing the outcomes of multiple STEP procedures. J Pediatr Surg 2017;52(1):69–73.
30. Cserni T, Takayasu H, Muzsnay Z, et al. New idea of intestinal lengthening and tailoring. Pediatr Surg Int 2011;27(9):1009–13.

31. Cserni T, Varga G, Erces D, et al. Spiral intestinal lengthening and tailoring - first in vivo study. J Pediatr Surg 2013;48(9):1907–13.
32. Cserni T, Biszku B, Guthy I, et al. The first clinical application of the spiral intestinal lengthening and tailoring (silt) in extreme short bowel syndrome. J Gastrointest Surg 2014;18(10):1852–7.
33. Alberti D, Boroni G, Giannotti G, et al. Spiral intestinal lenghtening and tailoring (SILT)" for a child with severely short bowel. Pediatr Surg Int 2014;30(11): 1169–72.
34. Coletta R, Aldeiri B, Morabito A. Institutional experience with spiral intestinal lengthening and tailoring. Eur J Pediatr Surg 2018 June 19. [Epub ahead of print]. https://doi.org/10.1055/s-0038-1660850.
35. Murphy F, Khalil BA, Gozzini S, et al. Controlled tissue expansion in the initial management of the short bowel state. World J Surg 2011;35(5):1142–5.
36. Collins J 3rd, Vicente Y, Georgeson K, et al. Partial intestinal obstruction induces substantial mucosal proliferation in the pig. J Pediatr Surg 1996;31(3):415–9.
37. Sudan D, Thompson J, Botha J, et al. Comparison of intestinal lengthening procedures for patients with short bowel syndrome. Ann Surg 2007;246(4):593–601 [discussion: 601–4].
38. Miyasaka EA, Brown PI, Teitelbaum DH. Redilation of bowel after intestinal lengthening proceduures – an indicator for poor outcome. J Pediatr Surg 2011;46(1): 145–9.
39. Jones BA, Hull MA, Potanos KM, et al. Report of 111 consecutive patients enrolled in the International Serial Transverse Enteroplasty (STEP) Data Registry: a retrospective observational study. J Am Coll Surg 2013;216(3):438–46.

Indications of Intestinal Transplantation

Arshad B. Kahn, MD, MS, MRCSed[a], Kiara A. Tulla, MD[b], Ivo G. Tzvetanov, MD[c],*

KEYWORDS

• Intestinal failure • Organ failure • Gastrointestinal anatomy

KEY POINTS

• The intestinal failure is the rarest form of organ failure that can arise from various conditions that affect gastrointestinal anatomy and function adversely.
• The management of this condition requires a multidisciplinary rehabilitation team with diverse experience to reduce complications and improve the longevity and quality of life.
• The role of autologous gastrointestinal reconstruction should be considered in patients with intestinal failure to promote enteral nutritional autonomy and wean off parenteral nutrition.
• Intestinal transplantation should be reserved for the patients with irreversible intestinal failure who develop life-threatening complications while on parenteral nutrition, with underlying life-threatening gastrointestinal disease.

INTRODUCTION

Permanent intestinal failure (IF) is the anatomic or functional reduction of the intestinal mass so that nutritional requirements for the fluids, macro- and micronutrients, are not met, leading to severe dehydration and malnutrition and inevitable death in the absence of any nutritional intervention. About 50% of adult patients with benign chronic IF can achieve enteral autonomy within the first 2 years. After that significant adaptation occurs in the minority, up to 94% of the adult patients have the probability of permanent IF requiring life-long PN.[1] Whereas in pediatric patients, intestinal adaptation and enteral autonomy can occur over a prolonged period in sharp contrast to adult.[2] Since its introduction, more than 50 years ago, parenteral nutrition (PN) is the gold standard of therapy for patients with benign chronic IF. From high morbidity and mortality in the past, PN has evolved significantly, and a recent series demonstrated that

Disclosure: None.
[a] Altru Health System, 715 Delmore Drive, Roseau, MN 56751, USA; [b] Department of Surgery, University of Illinois at Chicago, 840 South Wood Street, 376 CSN, M/C 958, Chicago, IL 60612, USA; [c] Division of Transplantation, Department of Surgery, University of Illinois at Chicago, 840 South Wood Street, Suite 402, Chicago, IL 60612, USA
* Corresponding author.
E-mail address: ltzveta@uic.edu

Gastroenterol Clin N Am 48 (2019) 575–583
https://doi.org/10.1016/j.gtc.2019.08.010
0889-8553/19/© 2019 Elsevier Inc. All rights reserved.

PN-dependent patients without complications and candidates of PN failure were able to achieve a 5-year survival of 87% and 73%, respectively.[3] Despite these advancements in PN, the PN-related complications are the most probable cause of death 2 years after the start of PN. Various series have demonstrated a complication rate of 19% to 26% in patients who are PN dependent.[3,4] The high rates of permanent IF after 2 years of total parenteral nutrition (TPN) coupled with high rate of PN-related complications in this window of time may lead to the selection of intestinal transplantation and other treatments, instead of PN in patients with permanent IF. Over these decades intestinal transplantation has emerged as an established and efficacious therapy for permanent IF. Most adult patients resume work and enjoy a good quality of life (QOL),[5] whereas most pediatric patients gain nutritional autonomy, catch up growth, and enjoy a good QOL.[6–8] The outcomes of intestinal transplantation have significantly improved. The latest intestinal transplant registry reveals 1-, 5-, and 10-year graft survival rates to be 71%, 50%, and 40% and the patient survival rates to be 77%, 58%, and 47%, respectively.[9] Despite the improved results of intestinal early transplantation currently in terms of comparable survival compared with home parenteral nutrition–dependent IF, a better QOL, and improved value of health care,[10–14] early transplantation has yet to become a standard of care.

CURRENT INDICATIONS OF THE INTESTINAL TRANSPLANTATION

Intestinal transplantation is reserved for patients with life-threatening complications of PN or underlying gastrointestinal disease.[15] Intestinal transplantation has emerged as a way to restore enteral autonomy in such patients. In the 2001 CMS memorandum, failure of PN therapy was defined by significant liver injury with elevated hepatic enzymes, multiple line infections, single episode of life-threatening catheter-related sepsis, thrombosis of 2 of the central veins, and frequent episodes of dehydration. These indications for intestinal transplantation approved by the Centers for Medicare and Medicaid Services for reimbursement[16] are listed in the following table.

FAILURE OF PARENTERAL NUTRITION

- Impending (total bilirubin 3–6 mg/dL, progressive thrombocytopenia, and progressive splenomegaly) or apparent liver failure (portal hypertension, hepatosplenomegaly, hepatic fibrosis, or cirrhosis) because of PN liver injury.
- Central venous catheter–related thrombosis of 2 central veins.
- Frequent central line sepsis: 2 episodes per year of systemic sepsis secondary to line infections requiring hospitalization; a single episode of line-related fungemia; septic shock; or acute respiratory distress syndrome.
- Frequent episodes of severe dehydration despite intravenous fluid in addition to PN.

The American Society of Transplantation proposed the following indications for intestinal transplantation in addition to the failure of PN[16,17]:
High risk of death attributable to the underlying disease.

- Desmoid tumors associated with familial adenomatous polyposis.
- Congenital mucosal disorders (eg, microvillus atrophy and intestinal epithelial dysplasia).
- Ultrashort bowel syndrome (gastrostomy, duodenostomy, residual small bowel 10 cm in infants and 20 cm in adults).

IF with high morbidity or low acceptance of PN.

- IF with high morbidity (frequent hospitalization, narcotic dependency) or inability to function (eg, pseudo-obstruction, high-output stoma).
- Patient's unwillingness to accept long-term PN (eg, young patients).

Still, other experts have suggested additional indications such as frozen abdomen, tumors of the mesenteric root, and complete portomesenteric thrombosis.[18]

Short bowel syndrome continues to be the leading underlying cause for IF and the referral cause for intestinal transplantation in 64% of the adults and 63% of the pediatric patients. The distribution of diseases underlying the indication for transplantation is age dependent. In children, these include gastroschisis (22%), volvulus (16%), enterocolitis (14%), atresia (4%), ischemia and trauma (1% each), and other causes (3%). The rest of the indications in children include motility disorders (18%), malabsorption (8%), tumors (1%), and retransplants (8%). In adults, IF is most frequently due to short bowel syndrome after extensive resections secondary to mesenteric ischemia (24%), inflammatory bowel disease (11%), small bowel tumors and tumors of the mesenteric root and retroperitoneum (13%), mobility disorders (11%), volvulus (8%), trauma (7%), and retransplantation (7%).[9]

INDICATIONS FOR TRANSPLANTATION OF DIFFERENT SMALL BOWEL CONTAINING ALLOGRAFTS

What defines intestinal transplantation is the implantation of a jejunoileal donor into a recipient. Depending on the inclusion of other organs along with the jejunoileum, intestinal transplantation can be classified into the following categories[19]:

1. Isolated intestinal transplantation (IITx) with or without a colon and pancreas or kidneys
2. Combined liver-intestine transplantation (LITx) with or without colon and or kidneys
3. Full multivisceral transplant (MVTx)—stomach, duodenum, pancreas, intestine, liver with colon, and kidney. Modified multivisceral transplant (MMVTx)—stomach, duodenum, pancreas, and intestine.

The choice of the allograft for a particular patient depends on several factors such as the cause of the permanent IF, presence of concurrent organ failure, availability of the donor organs, donor-recipient size match, the anatomy of the recipient, availability of the organs, and the experience of the transplant center.[20]

Isolated intestinal transplantation

IITx is indicated in patients with the IF that cannot be managed on total PN due to the failure of PN, high risk of death due to underlying disease, or high morbidity IF.[16,17] It is also indicated in patients with IF with mild to moderate liver dysfunction due to TPN before irreversible liver failure occurs.[21]

Right colon is included based on superior mesenteric artery with intestinal graft. The current colonic inclusion rate is 30%. The inclusion of colon did not adversely affect the survival, and colonic inclusion leads to a 5% higher rate of nutritional autonomy than those without the colon.[9] Moreover, colonic inclusion is associated with higher frequency of formed stools,[22] underscoring the important fact that ileocecal valve and the right colon enhance the gut function by better fluid absorption and fatty acid metabolism.[22–24]

The pancreas can be translated along with the intestine as a composite graft or a simultaneous pancreas and intestine transplantation from the same donor in patients with pancreatic insufficiency due to type 1 diabetes mellitus or cystic fibrosis.[20]

Concurrent evaluation for kidney transplantation should be considered in patients who are already on dialysis or those patients who have kidney dysfunction, as up to 20% of the patients after intestinal transplantation develop chronic renal failure.[25,26]

COMBINED LIVER-INTESTINE TRANSPLANTATION

Combined LITx is indicated in patients with IF and impeding or overt irreversible liver failure due to PN called as PN-associated liver disease (PNALD).[9,20,27–30] It is also indicated in patients with IF due to hypercoagulable state due to deficiency of protein C or S, which can be corrected by a liver graft.[31] The liver is transplanted en bloc along with the pancreas and small bowel. This avoids the hilar dissection and decreases the risk of biliary and vascular complications.[30] There is no clear consensus about when a liver should be included in the allograft. According to the intestinal transplant registry report, the inclusion of the liver in intestinal transplants declined to 48% between 2001 and 2011, reflecting the advances in the understanding of patients with PNALD and better management of patients on long-term PN.

Studies are rife with universal mortality at 5 years in patients with IF with cirrhosis in the absence of transplantation.[29,32] Another study revealed universal mortality at a median of 10.8 months following the first elevation of bilirubin in 6 patients with end-stage liver disease related to PN.[33] Based on these results it is accepted that combined LITx be offered to the patients with established cirrhosis or advanced fibrosis (stage III or IV fibrosis), whereas patients with early stage fibrosis should be offered intestine-only transplant, which by restoration of nutritional autonomy allows the gradual weaning and withdrawal of PN leading to resolution of PNALD.[20,34,35] Thus, it is mandatory that the patients with persistent elevation of bilirubin and low platelet count should undergo a transjugular biopsy to quantify the stage of fibrosis and portal pressure gradient in order to guide the type of allograft.

MULTIVISCERAL AND MODIFIED MULTIVISCERAL TRANSPLANTATION

MVTx is defined differently in different programs. In some centers MVTx is defined as transplantation of all organs supplied by celiac and superior mesenteric artery, viz, liver, stomach, duodenum, pancreas, and jejunoileal,[20,36] whereas the inclusion of stomach and duodenum along with jejunoileal is referred to as MVTx at other centers.[20,27] MVTx may be full if it involves the liver. Otherwise, it is called MMVTx.

Some investigators restrict the term MVTx to the allografts containing stomach,[10] whereas others include any combination of abdominal organs.

MVTx is offered to selected patients with portomesenteric thrombosis with hepatic decompensation, which is currently the most frequent indication.[20,27,28]

Other indications include the following: intraabdominal tumors that have led to local invasion require upper abdominal exenteration for a surgical cure and show no evidence for distant metastases,[37] familial polyposis syndromes, traumatic loss of abdominal viscera, and chronic intestinal pseudo-obstruction.[20,28] MMVTx excluding the liver is performed wherever the native liver function is preserved. The addition of the pancreas and duodenum in MVTx makes the surgery simple, as only a single-donor iliac Y-graft conduit to the recipient aorta is needed, the vena cava is replaced along with the liver, and no reconstruction of the porta hepatis is required, as the donor bile duct, arterial system, and portal vein remain intact, obviating the chances of biliary or arterial complications.[38]

POTENTIAL INDICATIONS OF SMALL BOWEL TRANSPLANTATION
Quality of Life Indications

With the improvement in outcomes of patients with intestinal transplantation, the QOL has become an important endpoint of intestinal transplantation. The ultimate aim of any therapeutic intervention is to alleviate the disease and improve the QOL. It has been well established that the QOL in recipients of intestinal transplantation is better than that in patients with IF on PN. Rovera and colleagues[39] reported a significant improvement in the QOL in the transplantation group compared with their pretransplant status when they were receiving PN. The most important finding, when comparing transplantation patients with a cohort of patients who were stable on PN, the QOL was similar between the 2 groups in spite of frequent complications in the immediate posttransplant period. Several other studies revealed that after intestinal transplant, children have physical and psychosocial functioning comparable to the normative population.[8,40] Similarly, many studies in adult intestinal transplant recipients have demonstrated improvement in many QOL domains, except depression and increased financial demands[41] in their peers on PN.[5,39,41–43] Furthermore, the largest report to date on QOL in adults and children with a follow-up of more than 2 decades revealed a higher rate of developmental, neurologic, and behavioral disorders among the visceral allograft recipients, particularly children. This was attributed to the effect of IF on early neuronal, emotional, and physical development, compounded by PN-associated complications with demonstrable pathologic changes in brain and various organs. These investigators recommended early consideration for transplantation in order to reduce these devastating, irreversible deficits particularly in children.[5] There is the caveat that this data are based on patients who are 1-year survivors, creating a bias on the effects of intestinal transplantation.

QOL as a potential indication for intestinal transplantation has not been approved by CMS, whereas the factors causing the unacceptable QOL, such as lethargy, pruritis, and hepatic osteodystrophy, are an established indication for liver transplantation. QOL is one of the primal advantages of intestinal transplantation compared with PN and hence should be considered as one of the potential indications for intestinal transplantation in the near future.

PSEUDOMYXOMA PERITONEI

Pseudomyxoma peritonei (PMP) is an uncommon slowly progressive condition that usually arises from perforation of appendix due to an enlarging appendiceal adenoma, allowing mucin-producing neoplastic cells to gain access to the peritoneal cavity.[44] Treatment involves cytoreductive surgery and heated intraperitoneal chemotherapy. However, disease recurrence can occur causing nutritional failure with extensive involvement of small bowel causing bowel obstruction and abdominal wall involvement with fistula formation. Reddy and colleagues[45] demonstrated in their series of patients with end-stage PMP, who underwent cytoreductive surgery followed by MVTx including abdominal wall transplantation (AWT), that such a procedure could restore nutritional autonomy, prolong life, and restore the excellent QOL.

ABDOMINAL WALL TRANSPLANTATION

One of the unique problems of IITx and MVTx patients is the small peritoneal space for the newly transplanted organs. This condition called as loss of domain results from loss of bowel due to multiple surgeries, fibrosis, scarring of the peritoneum, infectious complications, scarring of the abdominal wall due to multiple surgeries and ostomies, and visceral allograft tissue edema. This predisposes to suboptimal closure of the abdominal wall, which is of major concern. The quest for a solution to this unique challenge has led to several innovative solutions to enlarge the abdominal cavity and achieve safe closure. There are various methods to attempt closure ranging from component separation, pretransplant tissue expanders, and cellular dermal allograft, which requires well-vascularized abdominal wall tissue. Nonvascularized rectus fascia can be used in circumstances of good skin coverage but poor quality of underlying tissues. Sometimes the mesh or skin graft over the transplanted bowel is used as a bailout procedure when other options are not feasible due to the fibrotic, deformed, and unreconstructable abdominal wall, as well as loss of abdominal domain. In such a case, AWT has emerged as a novel option restoring a dynamic abdominal wall.[46]

The abdominal wall vascularized composite allograft is based on an inferior epigastric artery, which is implanted using the principles of direct orthotopic vascularization based on recipient's inferior epigastric or deep circumflex iliac artery. In simultaneous transplantation with intestine, no additional immunosuppression is required. The skin of the abdominal wall allograft may act as an immunomodulator, a sentinel marker for immunologic activity in the host, and a surrogate marker of rejection, allowing manifestation of the rejection to be seen on the visual inspection in the form of skin rash. In a study comparing IITx and MVTx with and without AWT, the investigators revealed that survival was similar in both groups (67% vs 61%); however, the AWT group showed faster posttransplant recovery, better intestinal graft survival (79% vs 60%), a lower intestinal rejection rate (7% vs 27%), and a lower rate of misdiagnoses in which viral infection was mistaken and treated as rejection (14% vs 33%).[47] Another study revealed that the rejection of AWT allograft might occur independent of small bowel rejection, but AWT rejection is a harbinger for subsequent small bowel rejection.[48,49] In their series of 5 patients, 2 patients developed AWT allograft rejection, which was recognized as a maculopapular rash without intestinal allograft rejection, which was treated successfully. One patient later developed a rash but did not seek medical attention leading to mild intestinal rejection underscoring the importance of early identification and treatment of skin rejection.[48] Since Levi and associates first introduced AWT, there have been 35 cases of abdominal wall allotransplants worldwide,[46] with 88% having flap survival.[50,51]

With the improvement in operative techniques and modern immunosuppression, the vascularized composite abdominal wall allografts could be used beyond visceral transplantation for complex abdominal wall reconstruction in nonvisceral transplant setting when other options are not feasible.

SUMMARY

Intestinal transplantation has made giant strides over the past few decades to the present era where current graft survivals are comparable with other solid organ transplants. The intestinal transplantation has been used primarily for patients with failure of PN or life-threatening underlying pathology. Given the better results, such restrictive indications should be lifted, and the intestinal transplantation should be offered to a broad cohort of patients with PN-dependent IF, as gut rehabilitation with the early restoration of nutritional autonomy has been shown to lead to improved survivals and better QOL.

REFERENCES

1. Messing B, Crenn P, Beau P, et al. Long-term survival and parenteral nutrition dependence in adult patients with the short bowel syndrome. Gastroenterology 1999;117(5):1043–50.

2. Spencer AU, Neaga A, West B, et al. Pediatric short bowel syndrome: redefining predictors of success. Ann Surg 2005;242(3):403–9 [discussion: 409–12].

3. Pironi L, Joly F, Forbes A, et al. Long-term follow-up of patients on home parenteral nutrition in Europe: implications for intestinal transplantation. Gut 2011;60(1):17–25.

4. Squires RH, Duggan C, Teitelbaum DH, et al. Natural history of pediatric intestinal failure: initial report from the Pediatric Intestinal Failure Consortium. J Pediatr 2012;161(4):723–8.e2.

5. Abu-Elmagd KM, Kosmach-Park B, Costa G, et al. Long-term survival, nutritional autonomy, and quality of life after intestinal and multivisceral transplantation. Ann Surg 2012;256(3):494–508.

6. Lacaille F, Vass N, Sauvat F, et al. Long-term outcome, growth and digestive function in children 2 to 18 years after intestinal transplantation. Gut 2008;57(4):455–61.

7. Sudan D, Horslen S, Botha J, et al. Quality of life after pediatric intestinal transplantation: the perception of pediatric recipients and their parents. Am J Transplant 2004;4(3):407–13.

8. Ngo KD, Farmer DG, McDiarmid SV, et al. Pediatric health-related quality of life after intestinal transplantation. Pediatr Transplant 2011;15(8):849–54.

9. Grant D, Abu-Elmagd K, Mazariegos G, et al. Intestinal transplant registry report: global activity and trends. Am J Transplant 2015;15(1):210–9.

10. Grant D, Abu-Elmagd K, Reyes J, et al. 2003 report of the intestine transplant registry: a new era has dawned. Ann Surg 2005;241(4):607–13.

11. Abu-Elmagd KM, Costa G, Bond GJ, et al. Five hundred intestinal and multivisceral transplantations at a single center: major advances with new challenges. Ann Surg 2009;250(4):567–81.

12. Abu-Elmagd KM. Intestinal transplantation for short bowel syndrome and gastrointestinal failure: current consensus, rewarding outcomes, and practical guidelines. Gastroenterology 2006;130(2 Suppl 1):S132–7.

13. Quintini C, Ward G, Shatnawei A, et al. Mortality of intra-abdominal desmoid tumors in patients with familial adenomatous polyposis: a single center review of 154 patients. Ann Surg 2012;255(3):511–6.

14. Abu-Elmagd KM, Reyes J, Fung JJ, et al. Evolution of clinical intestinal transplantation: improved outcome and cost effectiveness. Transplant Proc 1999;31(1–2):582–4.

15. Pironi L, Arends J, Bozzetti F, et al. ESPEN guidelines on chronic intestinal failure in adults. Clin Nutr 2016;35(2):247–307.

16. Buchman AL, Scolapio J, Fryer J. AGA technical review on short bowel syndrome and intestinal transplantation. Gastroenterology 2003;124(4):1111–34.

17. Kaufman SS, Atkinson JB, Bianchi A, et al. Indications for pediatric intestinal transplantation: a position paper of the American Society of Transplantation. Pediatr Transplant 2001;5(2):80–7.

18. Mangus RS, Tector AJ, Kubal CA, et al. Multivisceral transplantation: expanding indications and improving outcomes. J Gastrointest Surg 2013;17(1):179–86 [discussion: 186–7].

19. Abu-Elmagd KM. The small bowel contained allografts: existing and proposed nomenclature. Am J Transplant 2011;11(1):184–5.
20. Nickkholgh A, Contin P, Abu-Elmagd K, et al. Intestinal transplantation: review of operative techniques. Clin Transplant 2013;27(Suppl 25):56–65.
21. Lopushinsky SR, Fowler RA, Kulkarni GS, et al. The optimal timing of intestinal transplantation for children with intestinal failure: a Markov analysis. Ann Surg 2007;246(6):1092–9.
22. Kato T, Selvaggi G, Gaynor JJ, et al. Inclusion of donor colon and ileocecal valve in intestinal transplantation. Transplantation 2008;86(2):293–7.
23. Aghdassi E, Plapler H, Kurian R, et al. Colonic fermentation and nutritional recovery in rats with massive small bowel resection. Gastroenterology 1994;107(3): 637–42.
24. Goulet O, Auber F, Fourcade L, et al, editors. Intestinal transplantation including the colon in children. Transplantation proceedings. Helsinki: Elsevier Science Publishing Company, Inc; 2002.
25. Ojo AO, Held PJ, Port FK, et al. Chronic renal failure after transplantation of a nonrenal organ. N Engl J Med 2003;349(10):931–40.
26. Ruebner RL, Reese PP, Denburg MR, et al. End-stage kidney disease after pediatric nonrenal solid organ transplantation. Pediatrics 2013;132(5):e1319.
27. Fishbein TM. Intestinal transplantation. N Engl J Med 2009;361(10):998–1008.
28. Matarese LE, Costa G, Bond G, et al. Therapeutic efficacy of intestinal and multivisceral transplantation: survival and nutrition outcome. Nutr Clin Pract 2007; 22(5):474–81.
29. Buchman AL, Iyer K, Fryer J. Parenteral nutrition–associated liver disease and the role for isolated intestine and intestine/liver transplantation. Hepatology 2006; 43(1):9–19.
30. Sudan DL, Iyer KR, Deroover A, et al. A new technique for combined liver/small intestinal transplantation. Transplantation 2001;72(11):1846–8.
31. Grant D. Intestinal transplantation: 1997 report of the international registry. Intestinal Transplant Registry. Transplantation 1999;67(7):1061–4.
32. Fryer J, Pellar S, Ormond D, et al. Mortality in candidates waiting for combined liver-intestine transplants exceeds that for other candidates waiting for liver transplants. Liver Transplant 2003;9(7):748–53.
33. Chan S, McCowen KC, Bistrian BR, et al. Incidence, prognosis, and etiology of end-stage liver disease in patients receiving home total parenteral nutrition. Surgery 1999;126(1):28–34.
34. Fiel MI, Sauter B, Wu HS, et al. Regression of hepatic fibrosis after intestinal transplantation in total parenteral nutrition liver disease. Clin Gastroenterol Hepatol 2008;6(8):926–33.
35. Gotthardt DN, Gauss A, Zech U, et al. Indications for intestinal transplantation: recognizing the scope and limits of total parenteral nutrition. Clin Transplant 2013;27:49–55.
36. Fryer JP. The current status of intestinal transplantation. Curr Opin Organ Transplant 2008;13(3):266–72.
37. Alessiani M, Tzakis A, Todo S, et al. Assessment of five-year experience with abdominal organ cluster transplantation. J Am Coll Surg 1995;180(1):1–9.
38. Sudan D. The current state of intestine transplantation: indications, techniques, outcomes and challenges. Am J Transplant 2014;14(9):1976–84.
39. Rovera GM, DiMartini A, Schoen RE, et al. Quality of life of patients after intestinal transplantation. Transplantation 1998;66(9):1141–5.

40. Sudan D, Iyer K, Horslen S, et al. Assessment of quality of life after pediatric intestinal transplantation by parents and pediatric recipients using the child health questionnaire. Transplant Proc 2002;34(3):963–4.
41. Pironi L, Baxter JP, Lauro A, et al. Assessment of quality of life on home parenteral nutrition and after intestinal transplantation using treatment-specific questionnaires. Am J Transplant 2012;12(Suppl 4):S60–6.
42. O'Keefe SJ, Emerling M, Koritsky D, et al. Nutrition and quality of life following small intestinal transplantation. Am J Gastroenterol 2007;102(5):1093–100.
43. DiMartini A, Rovera GM, Graham TO, et al. Quality of life after small intestinal transplantation and among home parenteral nutrition patients. JPEN J Parenter Enteral Nutr 1998;22(6):357–62.
44. Khan AB, Al Suhaibani Y, Al Mohaimed K, et al. Application of advanced multimodality care to pseudomyxoma peritonei patient: report of first patient treated at a tertiary center. Indian J Surg Oncol 2010;1(3):270–3.
45. Reddy S, Cecil T, Allan P, et al. Extending the Indications of Intestinal Transplantation - modified multivisceral transplantation for end-stage pseudomyxoma peritoneii. Transplantation 2017;101(6S2):S89.
46. Park SH, Eun SC. Abdominal Wall Transplant Surgery. Exp Clin Transplant 2018; 16(6):745–50.
47. Gerlach UA, Vrakas G, Sawitzki B, et al. Abdominal wall transplantation: skin as a sentinel marker for rejection. Am J Transplant 2016;16(6):1892–900.
48. Allin BS, Ceresa CD, Issa F, et al. A single center experience of abdominal wall graft rejection after combined intestinal and abdominal wall transplantation. Am J Transplant 2013;13(8):2211–5.
49. Giele H, Vaidya A, Reddy S, et al. Current state of abdominal wall transplantation. Curr Opin Organ Transplant 2016;21(2):159–64.
50. Berli JU, Broyles JM, Lough D, et al. Current concepts and systematic review of vascularized composite allotransplantation of the abdominal wall. Clin Transplant 2013;27(6):781–9.
51. Lauro A, Vaidya A. Role of "reduced size" liver/bowel grafts in the "abdominal wall transplantation" era. World J Gastrointest Surg 2017;9(9):186–92.

Generating an Artificial Intestine for the Treatment of Short Bowel Syndrome

Mark L. Kovler, MD[a], David J. Hackam, MD, PhD[b],*

KEYWORDS

- Intestinal stem cells • Artificial intestine • Tissue engineering

KEY POINTS

- Intestinal failure remains a challenging clinical condition, and effective options for patients that fail to achieve enteral autonomy are limited.
- Recent advances in the ability to culture intestinal stem cells and cellular components of the enteric nervous system have increased understanding of the regenerative capacity of the intestine.
- A tissue-engineered small intestine derived from cultured stem cells is attainable, although ongoing challenges exist.

INTRODUCTION

Intestinal failure is defined as the inability to maintain fluid, nutrition, energy, and micronutrient balance that leads to malnutrition and dehydration.[1-3] Causes of intestinal failure include short bowel syndrome, which refers to the loss of intestinal length resulting in a reduction in absorptive surface area,[2,3] and chronic severe intestinal dysmotility, in which impaired peristalsis results in chronic functional obstruction, which reduces nutrient intake.[4] Specifically, short bowel syndrome–associated intestinal failure results from massive loss of intestinal length, frequently after a bowel resection performed for one of several reasons, including mesenteric ischemia, inflammatory bowel disease, volvulus, radiation enteritis, necrotizing enterocolitis (NEC), surgical complications, and trauma.[3,5] Other congenital anomalies, such as severe

Disclosure: No competing financial interests exist.
[a] Division of Pediatric Surgery, Johns Hopkins University, Johns Hopkins Children's Center, 1800 Orleans Street, Baltimore, MD 21287, USA; [b] Pediatrics and Cell Biology, Division of Pediatric Surgery, Johns Hopkins University School of Medicine, Johns Hopkins Children's Center, The Charlotte R. Bloomberg Children's Center, Johns Hopkins University, Suite 7323, 1800 Orleans Street, Baltimore, MD 21287, USA
* Corresponding author.
E-mail address: Dhackam1@jhmi.edu
twitter: @davidhackam (D.J.H.)

intestinal atresia and gastroschisis, can result in short bowel syndrome. In addition, intestinal failure can occur in the presence of preserved intestinal length as a result of severe gastrointestinal dysmotility. In the setting of chronic dysmotility, chronic, nonmechanical intestinal obstruction develops, resulting in (or from) segmental luminal dilatation, and bacterial overgrowth can ensue, leading to malabsorption and feeding intolerance.[4,6] Studies have shown that intestinal failure secondary to dysmotility can be more severe than short bowel syndrome–associated intestinal failure, with more difficulty weaning from parenteral nutrition.[4,6]

In the setting of intestinal failure, patients are provided with intravenous fluid and parenteral nutrition in order to provide nutrition, hydration, and electrolyte balance.[7] Further, in an effort to encourage adaptation of the existing intestine and to restore intestinal function, intestinal rehabilitation programs encourage functional compensation through careful management of diet, and the selected administration of hormone and growth factor supplementation.[8] However, even with maximal medical therapy, only approximately 45% to 65% of patients with short bowel syndrome–associated intestinal failure achieve long-term enteral autonomy.[9–13] For the others, long-term use of parenteral nutrition is costly and plagued with medical complications, including liver failure, ongoing electrolyte derangements, and sepsis associated with central line use.[14–18]

For those patients who do not achieve enteral autonomy and experience repeated complications of parenteral nutrition, surgical treatments for intestinal failure may be indicated. These operations include gastrointestinal reconstruction and intestinal transplant.[19,20] The 2 options for reconstruction of the native intestine are the longitudinal intestinal lengthening and tailoring (LILT) and serial transverse enteroplasty (STEP) procedures.[21,22] The purpose of both of these operations is to provide increased functional length and surface area for absorption and decrease segmental dilatation. The LILT technique was introduced by Bianchi[21] in 1980, and involves longitudinal division of the dilated intestinal lumen in order to form 2 equally sized lumens, which maintain their blood supply, and are subsequently anastomosed in an end-to-end fashion, thus doubling the original intestinal length. The STEP, introduced in 2003 by Kim and colleagues,[22] increases the surface area for absorption by the creation of serial partial transections of a dilated portion of intestine in a zigzag pattern. In appropriately selected patients, these operations can improve outcomes, but they are not universally successful.[23,24] Factors associated with successful surgical results include preserved preoperative liver function and longer bowel length[25–28]; however, even when the initial operation fails and recurrent dilation occurs, repeat STEP can be performed, although outcomes are worse.[29]

For a subset of patients with intestinal failure with refractory complications of parenteral nutrition, intestinal transplant may be an option. Although early attempts at intestinal transplant were met with poor outcomes, with increased experience at high-volume centers, outcomes are improving; the 1-year, 5-year, and 10-year survival rates for patients transplanted between 2007 and 2016 are reported to be 87%, 70%, and 67% respectively.[30] However, access to high-volume centers and the requirement for long-term immunosuppression remain challenges.[31–33]

Based on these results, the need persists for next-generation therapies for patients with intestinal failure. Harnessing the intestine's own capacity for regeneration and the creation of a tissue-engineered small intestine are novel remedies for this devastating condition. This article reviews the current understanding and recent developments in regenerative intestinal therapy with special attention to clinical applications for patients with intestinal failure.

INTESTINAL REGENERATION
Cell Biology and Physiology of the Intestinal Epithelium

The intestinal epithelium consists of 2 regions known as the crypt, at the base, and the villus, at the tip. The crypt-villus axis provides the architecture necessary for continuous proliferation and replacement of dying and damaged mature cells of the epithelium.[34] This structure is critical for the functional elements of the intestinal epithelium: absorption, protection, and secretion. The villi create a large surface area configuration, which maximizes absorptive capacity in the small intestine. In contrast, the crypts are sheltered from mechanical and chemical stress, which is important to the survival of the regenerative cells that reside there.[35] The cells of the crypt-villus axis and the discussed influences on intestinal stem cell activity are summarized in **Fig. 1**.

The villi are populated by differentiated cells that are either primarily absorptive or secretory based on function. The most abundant cell in the epithelium is the enterocyte, which is responsible for absorption and intestinal barrier function. Primarily secretory cells are goblet, enteroendocrine, and tuft cells.[36] Goblet cells are the most abundant secretory cells, and their product, mucin, plays a protective role for the intestinal epithelium. Enteroendocrine cells produce and secrete hormones that serve a wide variety of functions, including nutrient and microbial sensing, communication with the enteric nervous system and gut motility, and hunger and satiety.[37] In addition, tuft cells are chemical sensors that play a role in taste sensation and opioid secretion.[38] In the transition region between crypt and villus, a unique population of progenitor cells exist, known as transit amplifying cells, a subset of cells that are highly proliferative with the ability to differentiate into all the cells of the villi.[39]

At the base of the intestinal epithelium, forming an invagination into the lamina propria, lies the crypt of Lieberkuhn,[40] also known as the intestinal crypt, which serves as the repository of intestinal stem cells. Crypt base columnar (CBC) cells are intestinal stem cells with important roles in epithelial regeneration and proliferation.[35] CBC cells are identified by positivity of the G protein–coupled receptor Lgr5.[35] In 2007, Clevers and colleagues[41] used fluorescent tracing of Lgr5+ cells in the intestine to show that CBC cells are actively cycling, distinct from other cells of the crypt, and have the ability to generate multiple lineages with the capacity for self-renewal in both the small and large intestine.

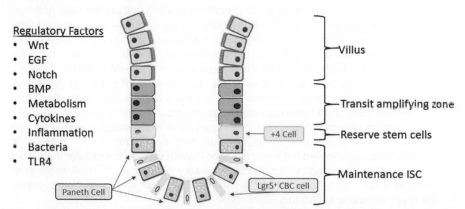

Regulatory Factors
- Wnt
- EGF
- Notch
- BMP
- Metabolism
- Cytokines
- Inflammation
- Bacteria
- TLR4

Villus

Transit amplifying zone

+4 Cell   Reserve stem cells

Maintenance ISC

Paneth Cell   Lgr5⁺ CBC cell

Fig. 1. Intestinal stem cell type, function and regulatory factors in the crypt-villus axis. BMP, bone morphogenetic protein; CBC, crypt base columnar; EGF, epidermal growth factor; ISC, intestinal stem cell; TLR4, Toll-like receptor 4.

Another self-renewing cell of the intestinal crypt is the so-called +4 cell, named for its position between the stem cell and progenitor cell zones of the crypt-villus axis.[35] These cells are marked by expression of the genes Bmi1, Hopx, mTert, and Lrig1.[42–45] The +4 cells contribute to intestinal regeneration under conditions of stress and injury, and thus have also been called reserve intestinal stem cells.[35]

In addition, the crypt contains differentiated cells in the form of Paneth cells and enteroendocrine cells. Paneth cells are differentiated cells that migrate downward as they differentiate, in the opposite direction to the villous differentiated cells, and thus are found entirely at the base of the crypt.[35] Paneth cells function to protect and influence their surrounding CBC stem cells. Through secretion of antimicrobial peptides, Paneth cells contribute to barrier protection.[46] Perhaps more importantly, Paneth cells provide molecular signals that regulate the functions of the intestinal stem cells through release of epidermal growth factor, Notch, and Wnt ligands, as discussed later.[35,46]

The Crypt-Villus Axis Response to Injury

Central to the development of novel therapeutic approaches to intestinal regeneration is an understanding of the crypt-villus axis in response to injury. Although homeostasis is maintained through the balance of epithelial cell loss and cell replacement under normal conditions, under conditions of damage or stress, significant plasticity of the intestinal epithelium in the form of redundant regenerative systems is necessary in order for it to undergo successful repair. In order for epithelial repair to be effective, a variety of intestinal progenitor cell subsets act in concert, including +4 stem cells, which serve as reserve stem cells.[35] Another subset of reserve stem cells that are active under stress are those expressing mouse telomerase reverse transcriptase (mTert).[44] These mTert+ cells are slow-cycling intestinal stem cells that can give rise to Lgr5+ cells as well as all differentiated intestinal cell types, and are resistant to radiation, unlike Lgr5+ and +4 intestinal stem cells.[44] In addition, differentiated lineage-committed epithelial cells have been shown to dedifferentiate and return to stemness, with Lgr5 positivity and the ability for both self-renewal and differentiation into other mature epithelial cell types.[47–49] Paneth cells also play a role in regulation of stem cells to increase proliferation and repair damage to the epithelium.[46]

Signaling Pathways in Intestinal Regeneration

Effective intestinal regeneration depends on intestinal stem cell proliferation and survival, which are regulated by the influence of several signaling pathways in the intestinal crypt. In a series of groundbreaking experiments published in 2009, Clevers and colleagues[50] were able to specify long-term culture conditions under which Lgr5+ stem cells could establish an ex vivo three-dimensional crypt-villus axis in the form of organoids. In doing so, they uncovered the components of the crypt niche that are necessary and sufficient for intestinal stem cell homeostasis. Although other crypt niche influences have since been described, the addition of only R-spondin (as a Wnt ligand), epidermal growth factor (EGF), and nogin (as a bone morphogenetic protein [BMP] inhibitor) were sufficient for crypt-villus axis development.[35,50] Further, in 2011, the same group showed the importance of Paneth cells as the cellular mediators of the intestinal crypt through which these regulatory signals act.[51] Thus, there exist both epithelial and mesenchymal influences on intestinal stem cell homeostasis, and the crypt structure allows this functionality.

As mentioned, the main epithelial influence comes from Paneth cells through the expression of Wnt, EGF, and Notch ligands.[52,53] Structurally, each crypt-based columnar cell is surrounded by Paneth cells, and the positioning of the CBC cells in relation to their neighboring Paneth cells determines their survival.[51,52] Through quantitative analysis of confetti-labeled Lgr5+ crypt-based columnar cells, Ritsma and colleagues[52] showed that positioning deep in the crypt, where CBC cells were surrounded by Paneth cells, led to a survival advantage, compared with at the edges of the crypt where Paneth cell contact was more limited. Additional support for the epithelial niche provided by Paneth cells is provided by experiments in which genetic Paneth cell (and their colonic counterpart) ablation led to reduction in crypt-based columnar cells.[51,54,55] Although epithelial support seems sufficient for intestinal stem cell survival, mesenchymal influences also have an impact by providing structural support and functional influence through Wnt, BMP, BMP antagonists, inflammatory cytokines, and endocrine factors.[35,56,57] Mechanistic understanding of the epithelial and mesenchymal influences on intestinal stem cells provides insight for novel therapies for intestinal failure, and the clinically relevant signaling pathways and their clinical applications are discussed later.

The Role of Wnt Signaling and Intestinal Regeneration

Wnt signaling is the most widely recognized pathway by which intestinal stem cell proliferation is regulated.[35] Wnt signaling in the intestinal crypt acts via Wnt ligand binding to Frizzled receptors, which inhibit degradation of cytoplasmic β-catenin, thus leading to β-catenin translocation to the nucleus and cell proliferation.[35,58] This process is critical under both normal and injury conditions, therefore it is an attractive target for therapeutic application.[59] The first intestinal organoids, a system described later, were developed from human Lgr5+ stem cells activated by the Wnt pathway.[50] With the potential for wide application to the treatment of patients with intestinal failure, our group has shown that activation of the receptor for gram-negative bacteria, namely Toll-like receptor 4 (TLR4), and also the inciting event in the pathogenesis of NEC (a common cause of intestinal failure in children), leads to impaired enterocyte proliferation through disruption of the Wnt–β-catenin pathway, and that restoration of this pathway can reduce the severity of NEC in mice through enhanced intestinal proliferation.[60] Wnt signaling has also been identified as a therapeutic target in other diseases, such as pancreatic and colon cancers, in which Wnt inhibition is attempted, and degenerative disorders such as congenital osteoporosis and Alzheimer disease.[58]

Functional Characteristics of Epidermal Growth Factor Signaling

EGF signaling through the ERBB1 receptor on crypt-based columnar cells increases intestinal stem cell proliferation.[35] EGF is produced by Paneth cells but also the underlying mesenchyme.[51] EGF plays a central role in enhancing intestinal organoid growth when added to its growth media and is readily soluble for administration, making it of therapeutic interest.[61] The role of EGF in intestinal adaptation and intestinal failure is well documented. In a mouse model of small bowel syndrome, Warner and Erwin[62] showed improved intestinal adaptation after stimulation of the EGF receptor. This finding was replicated in zebrafish, piglets, and rats.[63–65] Subsequent human studies of enteral treatment with EGF in patients with short bowel syndrome have shown promise.[66] Regarding prevention of short bowel syndrome, our group and others have shown the protective role of EGF signaling in attenuating NEC.[67,68]

Notch Signaling

Notch signaling acts through lateral inhibition between adjacent cells expressing Notch ligands (DLL1 or DLL4) and Notch receptors (NOTCH1).[35] In the intestinal crypt, Notch ligands are provided by Paneth cells, and restrict crypt-based columnar cell differentiation into a secretory lineage in order to maintain intestinal stem cell populations and appropriate cell ratios.[51] Notch signaling has been detected early after massive small bowel resection and is associated with increased proliferation of intestinal crypt epithelial cells.[69,70] Therefore, Notch signaling is an attractive target for therapies to treat intestinal failure in order to replenish the population of intestinal stem cells.

Bone Morphogenetic Protein in the Healing Response

BMP ligands (BMP2 and BMP4 in the intestine) are secreted by mesenchymal cells and promote cell differentiation.[71] BMP ligand secretion is controlled in a gradient along the intestinal villi by mesenchymal inhibition from myofibroblasts and smooth muscle cells.[71,72] After induction of short bowel syndrome by massive small bowel resection in rats, Coran and colleagues[73] showed increased BMP ligand expression in the later stages of intestinal adaptation, indicating the importance of cell differentiation 2 weeks after induction of the model.

A Role for Metabolism in Intestinal Regeneration

Emerging studies have highlighted the potential influence of metabolism on intestinal regeneration, which may have immediate clinical applications for patients with intestinal failure. Intestinal regeneration is an energy-intensive process, and metabolic conditions dependent on availability of nutrition may regulate the intestinal crypt stem cell activity.[35,74] Intestinal stem cells are highly reliant on mitochondrial activity and oxidative phosphorylation.[75] In contrast, differentiated cells of the intestinal epithelium depend predominately on glycolysis.[75] Therefore, energy states may dictate the ability for stem cell differentiation and proliferation. Although calorie restriction leads to mucosal atrophy, +4 stem cells are increased in number, providing a reserve system that can lead to increased intestinal epithelial regeneration when energy becomes abundant again.[76–78] In contrast, nutrient excess depletes Paneth cells, which in turn increases crypt-based columnar cell self-regeneration and may help elucidate the association between high-fat diets and intestinal cancers.[79,80] A better understanding of the role of nutrition and metabolism in intestinal failure could lead to optimization of this system to improve outcomes for patients immediately.

Stem Cell Therapy for Intestinal Failure

Given the rapid expansion in the understanding of intestinal stem cell physiology, application of stem cell–based therapy as a next-generation targeted and personalized treatment of patients with intestinal failure is ongoing. Although specific approaches to regenerate functional intestine after intestinal failure have not been established, several preclinical studies have shown promise in using stem cell therapies for the treatment of NEC, a common cause of short bowel syndrome in children.

NEC is a devastating disease of prematurity that usually develops after formula feeding in premature infants, and results in patchy intestinal ischemic necrosis.[81] Half of patients with NEC require surgery, and frequently extensive resection is necessary to remove the diseased bowel and cease the hyperinflammatory process. Intestinal failure secondary to short bowel syndrome in survivors is a common occurrence. Despite decades of research, effective therapies for treating NEC are lacking.[81] Several stem cell therapies have been attempted in animal models of the disease.[82] Zani and colleagues[83] delivered amniotic stem cells via intraperitoneal injection to rats induced with NEC and showed their integration into the bowel wall and improvement in survival and reduction in NEC severity. The mechanism for improvement was promotion of enterocyte proliferation through upregulation of Wnt–β-catenin signaling.[83] The benefits of amniotic fluid in NEC were subsequently shown to decrease disease severity by a decrease in TLR4 signaling and activation of the EGF and activation of the epidermal growth factor receptor (EGFR) by our group and others.[84,85] In a different approach, Besner and colleagues[86,87] found improvements in NEC with treatment derived from mesenchymal stem cells. Although direct stem cell–based therapies have not been effective in inducing native intestinal regeneration after intestinal failure, application of the knowledge gained on intestinal stem cells has led to the development of in vitro culture systems in the form of intestinal organoids, which show promise for patients with intestinal failure.

ORGANOID UNITS: THE BRIDGE FROM INTESTINAL REGENERATION TO THE DEVELOPMENT OF AN ARTIFICIAL GUT
Intestinal Organoid Units

The bridge between the understanding of intestinal regeneration and a therapeutic application of this knowledge toward the treatment of intestinal failure and short bowel syndrome lies in the ability to culture intestinal stem cells in three-dimensional units called organoids. Intestinal organoids are arrangements that contain the cellular diversity of native intestines, as described earlier, and can be cultured from primary tissue.[88] Clevers group embedded crypt derived cells in Matrigel and stimulated them with the niche elements described previously, resulting in three-dimensional structures with Lgr5+ and Paneth cells on the outside, and differentiated villous-like structures in the center.[50] The term organoid has been expanded to describe cell accumulations that are derived from different cell types, including exclusively epithelial cells, epithelial-mesenchymal tissue–derived combinations, and those derived from pluripotent stem cells.[88] Each approach has been completed with some success and replicated by our group and others (**Fig. 2**).[61,89–96] As mentioned, three-dimensional structures containing a progenitor-differentiated cell axis have been generated, but the initial structure did not closely resemble the crypt-villus axis that is necessary for proper intestinal regeneration.[97] In an effort to solve this issue, Sachs and colleagues[98] replaced Matrigel with type 1 collagen as the scaffold to support organoid cultures and were able to develop macroscopic tubal structures with an intact epithelium lining the inside, and cryptlike buds on the outer diameter. Further progress has been made using so-called designer matrices to support crypt-villus development.[99] Increased acceptance that development of a functional intestinal epithelium requires interaction with a complex immunologic and microbial environment has led to organoid growth in two-dimensional culture systems that permit separation of apical and basal conditions.[100,101]

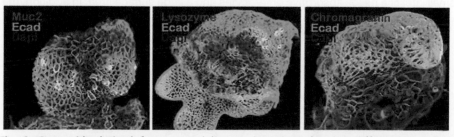

Fig. 2. Organoids derived from normal human intestine, showing differentiation into absorptive enterocytes (*green*), goblet cells (*red, left*), Paneth cells (*red, middle*), and enteroendocrine cells (*red, right*). Blue color for nuclear staining. (*Data from* Refs.[119])

Organoid-Based Therapy and Transplant

Organoid transplant has not yet been tested for restoration of intestinal function in an intestinal failure model, but success in animal models of colitis has shown promise. In a mouse model of dextran sulfate sodium–induced colitis, colonic organoids have been transplanted and subsequently integrated into the murine colon, which led to coverage of areas with mucosal damage and lack of intact epithelium.[90] This approach has led to improvement in weight gain in the mice, indicating that the engrafted organoids served in a functional absorptive capacity. Follow-up studies showed similar results using enteroids derived from fetal intestine and human tissue.[102,103] In a further step toward functional treatment, Helmrath and colleagues[93,104] transplanted human intestinal organoids from both intestinal and pluripotent stem cells into the mesentery of mice. The organoids develop a robust splanchnic blood supply. In a major technical achievement, they have successfully anastomosed these transplanted human intestinal organoids to the native mouse intestine.[105] Despite recent advances in organoid technology, the applications for short bowel syndrome and intestinal failure are limited by the inability to increase intestinal length and functional surface area, the goals of the tissue-engineered small intestine.

GENERATION OF AN ARTIFICIAL GUT: THE TISSUE-ENGINEERED SMALL INTESTINE
Tissue-Engineered Small Intestine

For patients with short bowel syndrome and intestinal failure who fail to achieve enteral autonomy through existing treatments, the development of a functional implantable intestine capable of nutrient absorption without the need for immunosuppression would be a lifesaving achievement. As with other tissue-engineered organs, the artificial intestine requires a source of progenitor cells and the necessary signals for regeneration, a tissue scaffold capable of housing the complex architecture of the intestine, and a mechanism of implantation and vascularization. An additional unique obstacle to attaining a tissue-engineered small intestine is the need for peristaltic motion.[106] Other obstacles to replacing the native intestine include the need to replace its endocrine and immunologic functions, although those functions do not seem to be necessary for the limited treatment of intestinal failure associated with short bowel syndrome.[107,108] Despite these challenges, the tissue-engineered small intestine is potentially achievable. The current status of the tissue-engineered small intestine is reviewed here, and breakthrough successes and opportunities for future discovery are highlighted (**Fig. 3**).

Cell Sources for Regenerative Proliferation

Epithelial lining
In order to meet the primary goal of enteral autonomy, a functional tissue-engineered small intestine needs absorptive enterocytes and a large surface area. In addition, the

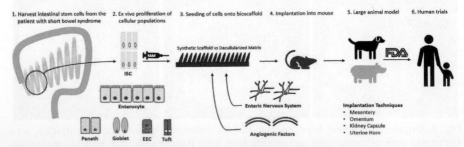

Fig. 3. Steps in the development of the tissue-engineered small intestine for the treatment of short bowel syndrome. EEC, enteroendocrine cell.

intestinal epithelium consists of several different cell types that play varying roles in secretion, defense, and communication. Although absorptive capability is paramount to the treatment of intestinal failure, it is likely that other differentiated cells of the intestinal epithelium (goblet cells, Paneth cells, enteroendocrine cells, tuft cells, and so forth; described earlier) contribute in essential ways to the overall function of the intestinal unit. Lgr5+ intestinal stem cells with and without mesenchymal components are capable of providing the regenerative capacity needed for a tissue-engineered mucosa, and the advances in organoid technology discussed earlier make this feasible.[50,61,89–91,109] Regarding the function of these units when implanted in vivo as a part of a tissue-engineered intestinal unit, the Grikscheit group has shown that, after 4 weeks, organoid units grown from both mice and humans and implanted into mice show both digestive and absorptive function.[110]

Mesenchymal components

The intestinal epithelium is sustained by a complex mesenchymal constituent that provides both structural support and functional influence. Myofibroblasts, macrophages, and smooth muscle cells all augment growth and differentiation of the intestinal epithelium, and contribute to native intestine function.[109,111,112] Incorporation of the native mesenchyme was first described in a tissue-engineered small intestine by Vacanti and colleagues[113] in a series of experiments in which organoid units on biodegradable scaffolds were implanted into the abdominal cavity of Lewis rats and wrapped in omentum before anastomosis with the native intestine, and subsequent examination showed the development of mesenchymal elements resembling native small intestine. After optimization of their polymer scaffold strategy, in 1999, the Vacanti group showed ingrowth of smooth muscle and fibrovascular tissue underlying the implanted tissue-engineered small intestine, which was augmented in the presence of an anastomosis between the native and tissue-engineered intestine.[114–116] Other groups have used embryonic and inducible pluripotent stem cells to produce both intestinal epithelium and surrounding mesenchyme.[117] Using the primary multicellular culture technique pioneered by Evans and colleagues,[118–120] our group and others have shown epithelial-mesenchyme integration on a tissue scaffold all of donor origin.

Tissue Scaffold

The construction of an appropriate tissue scaffold on which to implant the cellular components required for the development of an artificial gut is critical to a therapeutically applicable tissue-engineered small intestine. The ideal scaffold is firm enough to hold suture and maintain patency, but sufficiently flexible to accommodate neighboring structures and allow for peristalsis. The scaffold must be biocompatible and have a low immunogenic profile. In addition, it must be clinically feasible and easily implantable. These challenges have led to several bioavailable scaffolds for tissue-engineered small intestines.[121] Broadly, the 2 main strategies for the development of a tissue platform are the use of a synthetically generated scaffold and the use of naturally occurring material. Initial scaffolds for bioengineered organs were described by several groups, including Vacanti and colleagues,[113] Badylak and colleagues,[122] and Atala and colleagues,[123] with early success using synthetic and xenogeneic approaches. Further refinement of synthetic bioscaffolds specifically for small intestine has led to expanded success using polyglycolic acid (PGA)–derived variants, including the polylactic glycolic acid scaffold used in our laboratory.[96,119,124,125] Synthetic scaffolds are advantageous because they are customizable, and synthesis and replicability are reliable. However, synthetic scaffolds, like any synthetic implantable material, increase immunogenicity.

In comparison, naturally derived materials from which all cells are removed have also been used as tissue scaffolds for tissue-engineered small intestine.[126–128] Naturally derived scaffolds are less immunogenic but are limited by donor availability, and the decellularization process may lead to long-term performance issues.[126] Totonelli and colleagues[127] were able to successfully decellularize an entire rat small intestine using detergent-enzymatic treatment to create a natural intestinal scaffold. This technique allows maintenance of a vascular connection through the main mesenteric vessels, and conservation of the crypt-villus architecture on which organoids could grow.[128] Another naturally derived matrix has been developed using collagen and hyaluronic acid with some success.[129,130] The diversity of techniques and applications of tissue scaffolds makes comparison across laboratories and studies difficult. However, Besner and colleagues compared PGA, polycaprolactone (PCL), and collagen scaffolds in their construct of a tissue-engineered small intestine. PGA with poly-L-lactic acid (PLLA) coating had the optimal pore size, mechanical properties, degradation rates, and a similar architecture to native intestine, indicating that the PGA-PLLA–coated scaffold is the best current scaffold for tissue-engineered intestine.[121] The authors have had similar success in using polylactic glycolic acid scaffolds (Fig. 4).[119,124] Most recently, our group has applied the concept of functional tissue engineering to recreate the biomechanical, structural, and functional properties of the native small intestine in the development of novel intestinal scaffolds. Using polyglycerol sebacate, a biomaterial that has superior controllable degradation and mechanical properties, Ladd and colleagues[131] engineered a scaffold specifically suited for intestinal replacement, mimicking the microarchitecture and structural properties of native intestinal tissue.

Vascularization and Implantation

In order for the implanted cells of a tissue-engineered small intestine to maintain viability, and for the primary function of nutritional absorption, the graft must develop a blood supply. Vascularization of implanted organoid units was first reported by the Vacanti group.[113–115,132] Since then, the omentum and renal capsule have served as the conventional sites for engraftment.[96,116,132] Liu and colleagues[133] recently compared the success of various in vivo incubation sites, including the omentum, mesentery, uterine horn membrane, and abdominal wall and subcutaneous spaces. Wrapping the scaffold in vascularized membranes was more favorable, and the omentum served the additional benefit of ease with inline intestinal anastomosis.[133] Moreover, the addition of vascular endothelial growth factor and platelet-derived growth factor has improved large vessel vascularization.[134,135] These studies have shown that neovascularization is capable of sustaining the cells of a tissue-engineered small intestine at the capillary level, but whether this angiogenesis is functionally capable of delivering absorbed nutrients remains to be answered.

Implantation into the mesentery, as recently performed by the Helmrath and Besner groups, may be a superior site for absorptive purposes, because the blood supply derived from the mesentery is in line with the native enterohepatic circulation.[105,133] Another approach is the previously described decellularized intestinal scaffold method, in which the main vascular pedicle of the small intestine remains intact. Kitano and colleagues[136] used detergent-based perfusion to decellularize a scaffold, which they populated with pluripotent stem cells, maintaining the native vascular network. After heterotopic transplant via anastomosis of the superior mesenteric artery and superior mesenteric vein to the carotid artery and jugular vein, respectively, they showed absorption of glucose and fatty acids in vivo.[136]

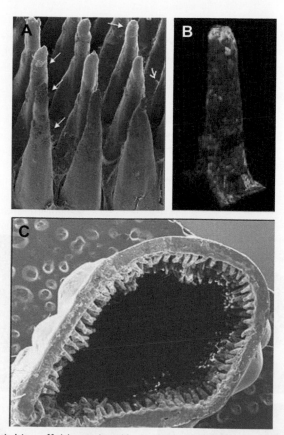

Fig. 4. (A) Synthetic bioscaffold populated by intestinal stem cells (*arrows*); (B) confocal scan of synthetic villus coated with differentiated epithelial cells; (C) tubularized intestinal scaffold before implantation. (*Data from* Shaffiey SA, Jia H, Keane T, et al. Intestinal stem cell growth and differentiation on a tubular scaffold with evaluation in small and large animals. *Regen Med.* 2016;11(1):45-61 and Costello CM, Hongpeng J, Shaffiey S, et al. Synthetic small intestinal scaffolds for improved studies of intestinal differentiation. *Biotechnol Bioeng.* 2014;111(6):1222-1232.)

Our group has similarly tested several methods of implantation in a newborn large animal model with long-term follow-up, assessing the feasibility of 3 clinically relevant models of implantation: a staged multioperation approach, a single-operation approach with defunctionalized loop-intestine graft, and a single-operation implantation with intestinal bypass (**Fig. 5**).[137] The single operation with intestinal bypass implantation had the fewest surgical complications.

The Enteric Nervous System and Peristaltic Motion in the Generation of an Artificial Intestine

Possibly the greatest challenge to a functional tissue-engineered small intestine is integration of the vast network of neurons and supporting cells that make up the enteric nervous system. The enteric nervous system, which is responsible for the coordinated movement of the intestine, is also active in secretion, taste, pain sensation, and crosstalk between the gut and the central nervous system. In achieving the development of a replacement enteric nervous system, neural tissue has been

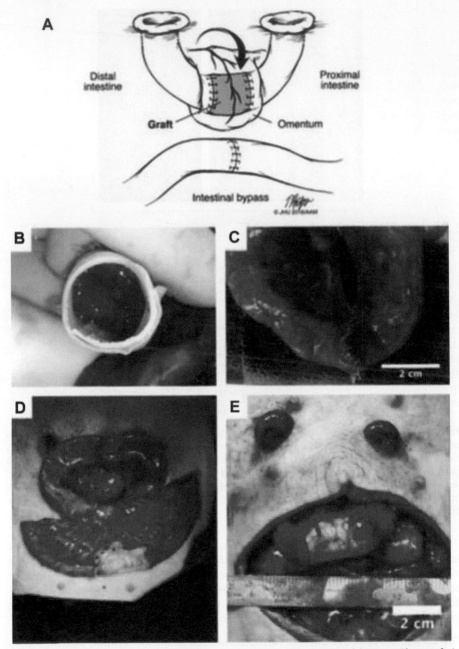

Fig. 5. (*A*) A single-operation implantation technique with intestinal bypass. The graft is anastomosed into a defunctionalized intestinal loop, which is brought to the skin with 2 mucous fistulas. (*B*) Graft anastomosis with the native intestine. (*C*) Primary anastomosis of the bypass segment of intestine. (*D*) Both the bypass and graft implantation completed, but before stoma maturation. (*E*) The ostomies matured through the abdominal wall and the omentum wrapped around the graft. (*From* Ladd MR, Martin LY, Werts A, et al. The Development of Newborn Porcine Models for Evaluation of Tissue-Engineered Small Intestine. *Tissue Eng Part C Methods.* 2018;24(6):331-345; with permission.)

cultured primarily from the intestine in the form of neurospheres, providing a cell source for the tissue-engineered small intestine.[138] Subsequently, the ability of human cultured neurospheres to populate aganglionic bowel has been shown by Goldstein and others in a model of Hirschsprung disease, supporting the ability to populate an aganglionic tissue-engineered small intestine with an enteric nervous system.[139–141] Most recently, murine neural progenitor cells derived from dorsal root ganglion have been used to generate an enteric nervous system in vivo.[142] Together, these studies emphasize the remarkable plasticity of neural progenitor cells and their ability to take residence and proliferate in aganglionic intestine. In 2017, Workman and colleagues[143] combined human pluripotent stem cell–derived neural crest cells with human intestinal organoids, and showed neuronal and glial activity, myenteric and submucosal plexus development, and integration with smooth muscle propagated contraction. Concurrently, the Grikscheit group achieved integration of a functional enteric nervous system on a human intestinal organoid tissue-engineered small intestine using enteric neural crest–derived neurospheres.[144] These advances indicate that establishment of an enteric nervous system and peristaltic motion are possible, overcoming maybe the greatest hurdle to a functional tissue-engineered small intestine.

SUMMARY

Intestinal failure from short bowel syndrome remains a challenging clinical condition, and the current options for patients that fail to achieve enteral autonomy through intestinal rehabilitation remain fraught with complications. Regenerative cell therapies and the tissue-engineered small intestine are novel next-generation strategies that have shown promise in other organ systems. However, the intestine is extremely complex, incorporating many different functions and critical cell types. Despite ongoing challenges, recent breakthroughs suggest that development of a functional, effective, and safe tissue-engineered small intestine is attainable.

REFERENCES

1. Belza C, Wales PW. Impact of multidisciplinary teams for management of intestinal failure in children. Curr Opin Pediatr 2017;29(3):334–9.
2. Buchman AL. Intestinal failure and rehabilitation. Gastroenterol Clin North Am 2018;47(2):327–40.
3. O'Keefe SJD, Buchman AL, Fishbein TM, et al. Short bowel syndrome and intestinal failure: Consensus definitions and overview. Clin Gastroenterol Hepatol 2006;4(1):6–10.
4. Vasant DH, Kalaiselvan R, Ablett J, et al. The chronic intestinal pseudo-obstruction subtype has prognostic significance in patients with severe gastrointestinal dysmotility related intestinal failure. Clin Nutr 2018;37(6):1967–75.
5. Batra A, Keys SC, Johnson MJ, et al. Epidemiology, management and outcome of ultrashort bowel syndrome in infancy. Arch Dis Child Fetal Neonatal Ed 2017; 102(6):F551–6.
6. Pakarinen MP, Kulvusalo AI, Rintala RJ. Outcomes of intestinal failure-a comparison between children with short bowel and dysmotile intestine. J Pediatr Surg 2009;44(11):2139–44.
7. Carroll RE, Benedetti E, Schowalter JP, et al. Management and complications of short bowel syndrome: an updated review. Curr Gastroenterol Rep 2016;18(7). https://doi.org/10.1007/s11894-016-0511-3.
8. Cisler JJ, Buchman AL. Intestinal adaptation in short bowel syndrome. J Investig Med 2005;53(8):402–13.

9. Infantino BJ, Mercer DF, Hobson BD, et al. Successful rehabilitation in pediatric ultrashort small bowel syndrome. J Pediatr 2013;163(5):1361–6.

10. Amiot A, Joly F, Lefevre JH, et al. Long-term outcome after extensive intestinal resection for chronic radiation enteritis. Dig Liver Dis 2013;45(2):110–4.

11. Demehri FR, Stephens L, Herrman E, et al. Enteral autonomy in pediatric short bowel syndrome: Predictive factors one year after diagnosis. J Pediatr Surg 2015;50(1):131–5.

12. Khan FA, Squires RH, Litman HJ, et al. Predictors of enteral autonomy in children with intestinal failure: a multicenter cohort study. J Pediatr 2015;167(1): 29–34.e1.

13. Modi BP, Langer M, Ching YA, et al. Improved survival in a multidisciplinary short bowel syndrome program. J Pediatr Surg 2008;43(1):20–4.

14. Kelly DA. Intestinal failure-associated liver disease: what do we know today? Gastroenterology 2006;130(2 SUPPL):70–7.

15. Moukarzel A, Haddad I, Ament M, et al. 230 patient years of experience with home long-term parenteral nutrition in childhood: natural history and life of central venous catheters. J Pediatr Surg 1994;29(10):1323–7.

16. Fonseca G, Burgermaster M, Larson E, et al. The relationship between parenteral nutrition and central line–associated bloodstream infections. JPEN J Parenter Enteral Nutr 2017;42(1). 014860711668843.

17. Barco S, Heuschen CBBCM, Salman B, et al. Home parenteral nutrition-associated thromboembolic and bleeding events: results of a cohort study of 236 individuals. J Thromb Haemost 2016;14(7):1364–73.

18. Gonzalez-Hernandez J, Daoud Y, Styers J, et al. Central venous thrombosis in children with intestinal failure on long-term parenteral nutrition. J Pediatr Surg 2016;51(5):790–3.

19. Rege AS, Sudan DL. Autologous gastrointestinal reconstruction: review of the optimal nontransplant surgical options for adults and children with short bowel syndrome. Nutr Clin Pract 2013;28(1):65–74.

20. Kesseli S, Sudan D. Small bowel transplantation. Surg Clin North Am 2019; 99(1):103–16.

21. Bianchi A. Intestinal loop lengthening-a technique for increasing small intestinal length. J Pediatr Surg 1980;15(2):145–51.

22. Kim HB, Fauza D, Garza J, et al. Serial transverse enteroplasty (STEP): a novel bowel lengthening procedure. J Pediatr Surg 2003;38:425–9.

23. King B, Carlson G, Khalil BA, et al. Intestinal bowel lengthening in children with short bowel syndrome: Systematic review of the Bianchi and STEP procedures. World J Surg 2013;37(3):694–704.

24. Javid PJ, Heung BK, Duggan CP, et al. Serial transverse enteroplasty is associated with successful short-term outcomes in infants with short bowel syndrome. J Pediatr Surg 2005;40(6):1019–24.

25. Jones BA, Hull MA, Potanos KM, et al. Report of 111 consecutive patients enrolled in the international serial transverse enteroplasty (STEP) data registry: a retrospective observational study. J Am Coll Surg 2013;216(3):438–46.

26. Oliveira C, De Silva N, Wales PW. Five-year outcomes after serial transverse enteroplasty in children with short bowel syndrome. J Pediatr Surg 2012;47(5): 931–7.

27. Javid PJ, Sanchez SE, Horslen SP, et al. Intestinal lengthening and nutritional outcomes in children with short bowel syndrome. Am J Surg 2013;205(5): 576–80.

28. Sommovilla J, Warner BW. Surgical options to enhance intestinal function in patients with short bowel syndrome. Curr Opin Pediatr 2014;26(3):350–5.

29. Piper H, Modi BP, Kim HB, et al. The second STEP: the feasibility of repeat serial transverse enteroplasty. J Pediatr Surg 2006;41(12):1951–6.

30. Venick RS. Long-term results of intestinal transplantation in children: survival after 10 years, intestinal function, quality of life. Curr Opin Organ Transpl 2018. https://doi.org/10.1097/MOT.0000000000000514.

31. Tzakis AG, Kato T, Levi DM, et al. 100 Multivisceral transplants at a single center. Ann Surg 2005;242(4):480–93.

32. Farmer DG, Venick RS, Colangelo J, et al. Pretransplant predictors of survival after intestinal transplantation: Analysis of a single-center experience of more than 100 transplants. Transplantation 2010;90(12):1574–80.

33. Beduschi T, Garcia J, Faag A, et al. Breaking the 5 year mark with 100% survival for intestinal transplant -time to become protagonist in the management of intestinal failure? Transplantation 2017;101. https://doi.org/10.1097/HJH.0000000000001787.

34. Darwich AS, Aslam U, Ashcroft DM, et al. Meta-analysis of the turnover of intestinal epithelia in preclinical animal species and humans. Drug Metab Dispos 2014;42(12):2016–22.

35. Gehart H, Clevers H. Tales from the crypt: new insights into intestinal stem cells. Nat Rev Gastroenterol Hepatol 2019;16:19–34.

36. Grosse AS, Pressprich MF, Curley LB, et al. Cell dynamics in fetal intestinal epithelium: implications for intestinal growth and morphogenesis. J Cell Sci 2011;124(20):e1.

37. Moran GW, Leslie FC, Levison SE, et al. Review: enteroendocrine cells: neglected players in gastrointestinal disorders? Therap Adv Gastroenterol 2008;1(1):51–60.

38. Gerbe F, Legraverend C, Jay P. The intestinal epithelium tuft cells: specification and function. Cell Mol Life Sci 2012;69(17):2907-17.

39. Hong AW, Meng Z, Guan KL. The Hippo pathway in intestinal regeneration and disease. Nat Rev Gastroenterol Hepatol 2016;13(6):324–37.

40. Clevers H. The intestinal crypt, a prototype stem cell compartment. Cell 2013;154(2):274.

41. Barker N, Van Es JH, Kuipers J, et al. Identification of stem cells in small intestine and colon by marker gene Lgr5. Nature 2007;449(7165):1003–7.

42. Sangiorgi E, Capecchi MR. Bmi1 is expressed in vivo in intestinal stem cells. Nat Genet 2008;40(7):915–20.

43. Takeda N, Jain R, LeBoeuf M, et al. Interconversion between intestinal stem cell populations in distinct niches. Science 2011;334:1420–4.

44. Montgomery RK, Carlone DL, Richmond CA, et al. Mouse telomerase reverse transcriptase (mTert) expression marks slowly cycling intestinal stem cells. Proc Natl Acad Sci U S A 2011;108(1):170–84.

45. Powell AF, Wang Y, Li Y, et al. The pan-ErbB negative regulator Irig1 is an intestinal stem cell marker that functions as a tumor suppressor. Cell 2012;149(1):146–58.

46. Gassler N. Paneth cells in intestinal physiology and pathophysiology. World J Gastrointest Pathophysiol 2017;8(4):150–60.

47. Yan KS, Gevaert O, Zheng GXY, et al. Intestinal enteroendocrine lineage cells possess homeostatic and injury-inducible stem cell activity. Cell Stem Cell 2017;21(1):78-90.e6.

48. Van Es JH, Sato T, Van De Wetering M, et al. Dll1 + secretory progenitor cells revert to stem cells upon crypt damage. Nat Cell Biol 2012;14(10):1099–104.

49. Tetteh PW, Basak O, Farin HF, et al. Replacement of lost Lgr5-positive stem cells through plasticity of their enterocyte-lineage daughters. Cell Stem Cell 2016; 18(2):203–13.

50. Sato T, Vries RG, Snippert HJ, et al. Single Lgr5 stem cells build crypt-villus structures in vitro without a mesenchymal niche. Nature 2009;459(7244):262–5.

51. Sato T, Van Es JH, Snippert HJ, et al. Paneth cells constitute the niche for Lgr5 stem cells in intestinal crypts. Nature 2011;469(7330):415–8.

52. Ritsma L, Ellenbroek SIJ, Zomer A, et al. Intestinal crypt homeostasis revealed at single-stem-cell level by in vivo live imaging. Nature 2014;507(7492):362–5.

53. Clevers HC, Bevins CL. Paneth cells: maestros of the small intestinal crypts. Annu Rev Physiol 2013;75(1):289–311.

54. Sasaki N, Sachs N, Wiebrands K, et al. Reg4 + deep crypt secretory cells function as epithelial niche for Lgr5 + stem cells in colon. Proc Natl Acad Sci U S A 2016;113(37):E5399–407.

55. Bastide P, Darido C, Pannequin J, et al. Sox9 regulates cell proliferation and is required for Paneth cell differentiation in the intestinal epithelium. J Cell Biol 2007;178(4):635–48.

56. Valenta T, Degirmenci B, Moor AE, et al. Wnt ligands secreted by subepithelial mesenchymal cells are essential for the survival of intestinal stem cells and gut homeostasis. Cell Rep 2016;15(5):911–8.

57. Stzepourginski I, Nigro G, Jacob J-M, et al. CD34 + mesenchymal cells are a major component of the intestinal stem cells niche at homeostasis and after injury. Proc Natl Acad Sci U S A 2017;114(4):E506–13.

58. Nusse R, Clevers H. Wnt/β-catenin signaling, disease, and emerging therapeutic modalities. Cell 2017;169(6):985–99.

59. Miyoshi H, Ajimma R, Luo C, et al. Wnt5a potentiates TGF-b signaling to promote colonic crypt regeneration after tissue injury. Science 2012;338:108–13.

60. Sodhi CP, Shi XH, Richardson WM, et al. Toll-like receptor-4 inhibits enterocyte proliferation via impaired β-catenin signaling in necrotizing enterocolitis. Gastroenterology 2010;138(1):185–96.

61. Sato T, Stange DE, Ferrante M, et al. Long-term expansion of epithelial organoids from human colon, adenoma, adenocarcinoma, and Barrett's epithelium. Gastroenterology 2011;141(5):1762–72.

62. Warner BW, Erwin CR. Critical roles for EGF receptor signaling during resection-induced intestinal adaptation. J Pediatr Gastroenterol Nutr 2006;43(1 SUPPL. 1): 68–73.

63. Schall KA, Holoyda KA, Grant CN, et al. Adult zebrafish intestine resection: a novel model of short bowel syndrome, adaptation, and intestinal stem cell regeneration. Am J Physiol Liver Physiol 2015;309(3):G135–45.

64. Lim DW, Levesque CL, Vine DF, et al. Synergy of glucagon-like peptide-2 and epidermal growth factor coadministration on intestinal adaptation in neonatal piglets with short bowel syndrome. Am J Physiol Liver Physiol 2017;312(4): G390–404.

65. Sham J, Martin G, Meddings JB, et al. Epidermal growth factor improves nutritional outcome in a rat model of short bowel syndrome. J Pediatr Surg 2002; 37(5):765–9.

66. Sigalet DL, Martin GR, Butzner JD, et al. A pilot study of the use of epidermal growth factor in pediatric short bowel syndrome. J Pediatr Surg 2005;40(5): 763–8.

67. Good M, Sodhi CP, Egan CE, et al. Breast milk protects against the development of necrotizing enterocolitis through inhibition of Toll Like Receptor 4 in the intestinal epithelium via activation of the epidermal growth factor receptor. Mucosal Immunol 2009;24(45):6848–54.

68. Wei J, Zhou Y, Besner GE. Heparin-binding EGF-like growth factor and enteric neural stem cell transplantation in the prevention of experimental necrotizing enterocolitis in mice. Pediatr Res 2015;78(1):29–37.

69. Chen G, Sun L, Yu M, et al. The jagged-1/Notch-1/Hes-1 pathway is involved in intestinal adaptation in a massive small bowel resection rat model. Dig Dis Sci 2013;58(9):2478–86.

70. Sukhotnik I, Dorfman T, Halabi S, et al. Accelerated intestinal epithelial cell turnover after bowel resection in a rat is correlated with inhibited hedgehog signaling cascade. Pediatr Surg Int 2016;32(12):1133–40.

71. Kosinski C, Li VSW, Chan ASY, et al. Gene expression patterns of human colon tops and basal crypts and BMP antagonists as intestinal stem cell niche factors. Proc Natl Acad Sci U S A 2007;104(39):15418–23.

72. He XC, Zhang J, Tong WG, et al. BMP signaling inhibits intestinal stem cell self-renewal through suppression of Wnt-β-catenin signaling. Nat Genet 2004; 36(10):1117–21.

73. Sukhotnik I, Berkowitz D, Dorfman T, et al. The role of the BMP signaling cascade in regulation of stem cell activity following massive small bowel resection in a rat. Pediatr Surg Int 2016;32(2):169–74.

74. Alonso S, Yilmaz ÖH. Nutritional regulation of intestinal stem cells. Annu Rev Nutr 2018;38(1):273–301.

75. Rodríguez-Colman MJ, Schewe M, Meerlo M, et al. Interplay between metabolic identities in the intestinal crypt supports stem cell function. Nature 2017; 543(7645):424–7.

76. Chappell VL, Thompson MD, Jeschke MG, et al. Effects of incremental starvation on gut mucosa. Dig Dis Sci 2003;48(4):765–9.

77. Richmond CA, Shah MS, Deary LT, et al. Dormant intestinal stem cells are regulated by pten and nutritional status. Cell Rep 2015;13(11):2403–11.

78. Yousefi M, Nakauka-Dbamba A, Berry CT, et al. Calorie restriction governs intestinal epithelial regeneration through cell-autonomous regulation of mTORC1 in reserve stem cells. Stem Cell Reports 2018;10(3):703–11.

79. Beyaz S, Mana MD, Roper J, et al. High-fat diet enhances stemness and tumorigenicity of intestinal progenitors. Nature 2016;531(7592):53–8.

80. Bardou M, Barkun AN, Martel M. Obesity and colorectal cancer. Gut 2013;62: 933–47.

81. Hackam DJ, Sodhi CP, Good M. New insights into necrotizing enterocolitis: from laboratory observation to personalized prevention and treatment. J Pediatr Surg 2019. https://doi.org/10.1016/j.jpedsurg.2018.06.012.

82. McCulloh CJ, Olson JK, Zhou Y, et al. Stem cells and necrotizing enterocolitis: a direct comparison of the efficacy of multiple types of stem cells. J Pediatr Surg 2017;52(6):999–1005.

83. Zani A, Cananzi M, Fascetti-Leon F, et al. Amniotic fluid stem cells improve survival and enhance repair of damaged intestine in necrotising enterocolitis via a COX-2 dependent mechanism. Gut 2014;63(2):300–9.

84. Good M, Siggers RH, Sodhi CP, et al. Amniotic fluid inhibits Toll-like receptor 4 signaling in the fetal and neonatal intestinal epithelium. Proc Natl Acad Sci U S A 2012;109(28):11330–5.

85. Siggers J, Østergaard MV, Siggers RH, et al. Postnatal amniotic fluid intake reduces gut inflammatory responses and necrotizing enterocolitis in preterm neonates. Am J Physiol Liver Physiol 2013;304(10):G864–75.

86. Rager TM, Olson JK, Zhou Y, et al. Exosomes secreted from bone marrow-derived mesenchymal stem cells protect the intestines from experimental necrotizing enterocolitis. J Pediatr Surg 2016;51(6):942–7.

87. Yang J, Watkins D, Chen CL, et al. Heparin-binding epidermal growth factor-like growth factor and mesenchymal stem cells act synergistically to prevent experimental necrotizing enterocolitis. J Am Coll Surg 2012;215(4):534–45.

88. Dedhia PH, Bertaux-Skeirik N, Zavros Y, et al. Organoid models of human gastrointestinal development and disease. Gastroenterology 2016;150(5): 1098–112.

89. Jung P, Sato T, Merlos-Suárez A, et al. Isolation and in vitro expansion of human colonic stem cells. Nat Med 2011;17(10):1225–7.

90. Yui S, Nakamura T, Sato T, et al. Functional engraftment of colon epithelium expanded in vitro from a single adult Lgr5 + stem cell. Nat Med 2012;18(4): 618–23.

91. Ootani A, Li X, Sangiorgi E, et al. Sustained in vitro intestinal epithelial culture within a Wnt-dependent stem cell niche. Nat Med 2009;15(6):701–6.

92. Li X, Nadauld L, Ootani A, et al. Oncogenic transformation of diverse gastrointestinal tissues in primary organoid culture. Nat Med 2014;20(7):769–77.

93. Watson CL, Mahe MM, Múnera J, et al. An in vivo model of human small intestine using pluripotent stem cells. Nat Med 2014;20(11):1310–4.

94. Mccracken KW, Howell JC, Wells JM, et al. Generating human intestinal tissue from pluripotent stem cells in vitro. Nat Protoc 2014;6(12):1920–8.

95. Aurora M, Spence JR. hPSC-derived lung and intestinal organoids as models of human fetal tissue. Dev Biol 2016;420(2):230–8.

96. Finkbeiner SR, Freeman JJ, Wieck MM, et al. Generation of tissue-engineered small intestine using embryonic stem cell-derived human intestinal organoids. Biol Open 2015;4(11):1462–72.

97. Nakamura T, Sato T. Advancing intestinal organoid technology toward regenerative medicine. Cell Mol Gastroenterol Hepatol 2018;5(1):51–60.

98. Sachs N, Tsukamoto Y, Kujala P, et al. Intestinal epithelial organoids fuse to form self-organizing tubes in floating collagen gels. Development 2017;144(6): 1107–12.

99. Gjorevski N, Sachs N, Manfrin A, et al. Designer matrices for intestinal stem cell and organoid culture. Nature 2016;539(7630):560–4.

100. Moon C, Vandussen KL, Miyoshi H, et al. Development of a primary mouse intestinal epithelial cell monolayer culture system to evaluate factors that modulate IgA transcytosis. Mucosal Immunol 2014;7(4):818–28.

101. VanDussen KL, Marinshaw JM, Shaikh N, et al. Development of an enhanced human gastrointestinal epithelial culture system to facilitate patient-based assays. Gut 2015;64(6):911–20.

102. Fordham RP, Yui S, Hannan NRF, et al. Transplantation of expanded fetal intestinal progenitors contributes to colon regeneration after injury. Cell Stem Cell 2013;13(6):734–44.

103. Sugimoto S, Ohta Y, Fujii M, et al. Reconstruction of the human colon epithelium in vivo. Cell Stem Cell 2018;22(2):171–6.e5.

104. Mahe MM, Sundaram N, Watson CL, et al. Establishment of human epithelial enteroids and colonoids from whole tissue and biopsy. J Vis Exp 2015; 97(97):1–13.

105. Cortez AR, Poling HM, Brown NE, et al. Transplantation of human intestinal organoids into the mouse mesentery: a more physiologic and anatomic engraftment site. Surgery 2018;164(4):643–50.

106. Dunn JCY. Is the tissue-engineered intestine clinically viable? Nat Clin Pract Gastroenterol Hepatol 2008;5(7):366–7.

107. Ladd MR, Niño DF, March JC, et al. Generation of an artificial intestine for the management of short bowel syndrome. Curr Opin Organ Transpl 2016;21(2): 178–85.

108. Martin LY, Ladd MR, Werts A, et al. Tissue engineering for the treatment of short bowel syndrome in children. Pediatr Res 2018;83(1–2):249–57.

109. Lei NY, Jabaji Z, Wang J, et al. Intestinal subepithelial myofibroblasts support the growth of intestinal epithelial stem cells. PLoS One 2014;9(1). https://doi.org/10.1371/journal.pone.0084651.

110. Grant CN, Mojica SG, Sala FG, et al. Human and mouse tissue-engineered small intestine both demonstrate digestive and absorptive function. Am J Physiol Liver Physiol 2015;308(8):G664–77.

111. Lahar N, Lei NY, Wang J, et al. Intestinal subepithelial myofibroblasts support in vitro and in vivo growth of human small intestinal epithelium. PLoS One 2011;6(11):1–9.

112. Graham HK, Maina I, Goldstein AM, et al. Intestinal smooth muscle is required for patterning the enteric nervous system. J Anat 2017;230(4):567–74.

113. Vacanti JP, Morse MA, Saltzman WM, et al. Selective cell transplantation using bioabsorbable artificial polymers as matrices. J Pediatr Surg 1988;23(1):3–9.

114. Choi RS, Vacanti JP. Preliminary studies of tissue-engineered intestine using isolated epithelial organoid units on tubular synthetic biodegradable scaffolds. Transplant Proc 1997;29(1–2):848–51.

115. Stephen KS, Kaihara S, Benvenuto MS, et al. Effects of anastomosis of tissue-engineered neointestine to native small bowel. J Surg Res 1999;87(1):6–13.

116. Grikscheit TC, Siddique A, Ochoa ER, et al. Tissue-engineered small intestine improves recovery after massive small bowel resection. Ann Surg 2004; 240(5):748–54.

117. Spence JR, Mayhew CN, Rankin SA, et al. Directed differentiation of human pluripotent stem cells into intestinal tissue in vitro. Nature 2011;470(7332): 105–10.

118. Liu Y, Terrence R, Johnson J, et al. Enriched intestinal stem cell seeding improves the architecture of tissue-engineered intestine. Tissue Eng Part C Methods 2015;21(8):816–25.

119. Shaffiey SA, Jia H, Keane T, et al. Intestinal stem cell growth and differentiation on a tubular scaffold with evaluation in small and large animals. Regen Med 2016;11(1):45–61.

120. Sala FG, Matthews JA, Speer AL, et al. A multicellular approach forms a significant amount of tissue-engineered small intestine in the mouse. Tissue Eng Part A 2011;17(13–14):1841–50.

121. Liu Y, Nelson T, Chakrott J, et al. Comparison of polyglycolic acid, polycaprolactone, and collagen as scaffolds for the production of tissue engineered intestine. J Biomed Mater Res B Appl Biomater 2018;1–11. https://doi.org/10.1002/jbm.b.34169.

122. Badylak SF. Xenogeneic extracellular matrix as a scaffold for tissue reconstruction. Transpl Immunol 2004;12(3–4):367–77.

123. Atala A, Bauer SB, Soker S, et al. Tissue-engineered autologous bladders for patients needing cystoplasty. Lancet 2006;367(9518):1241–6.

124. Costello CM, Hongpeng J, Shaffiey S, et al. Synthetic small intestinal scaffolds for improved studies of intestinal differentiation. Biotechnol Bioeng 2014;111(6): 1222–32.

125. Liu Y, Nelson T, Cromeens B, et al. HB-EGF embedded in PGA/PLLA scaffolds via subcritical CO_2 augments the production of tissue engineered intestine. Biomaterials 2016;103:150–9.

126. Del Gaudio C, Ajalloueian F, Baiguera S, et al. Are synthetic scaffolds suitable for the development of clinical tissue-engineered tubular organs? J Biomed Mater Res A 2013;102(7):2427–47.

127. Totonelli G, Maghsoudlou P, Garriboli M, et al. A rat decellularized small bowel scaffold that preserves villus-crypt architecture for intestinal regeneration. Biomaterials 2012;33(12):3401–10.

128. Maghsoudlou P, Totonelli G, Loukogeorgakis SP, et al. A decellularization methodology for the production of a natural acellular intestinal matrix. J Vis Exp 2013;(80):1–6.

129. Nakase Y, Hagiwara A, Nakamura T, et al. Tissue engineering of small intestinal tissue using collagen sponge scaffolds seeded with smooth muscle cells. Tissue Eng 2006;12(2):403–12.

130. Sung JH, Yu J, Luo D, et al. Microscale 3-D hydrogel scaffold for biomimetic gastrointestinal (GI) tract model. Lab Chip 2011;11(3):389–92.

131. Ladd MR, Costello C, Gosztyla C, et al. Development of intestinal scaffolds that mimic native mammalian intestinal tissue. Tissue Eng Part A 2019;1–45. https://doi.org/10.1089/ten.tea.2018.0239.

132. Gardner-Thorpe J, Grikscheit T, Ito H, et al. Angiogenesis in tissue-engineered small intestine. Tissue Eng 2003;9(6):1255–61.

133. Liu Y, Cromeens BP, Wang Y, et al. Comparison of different in vivo incubation sites to produce tissue-engineered small intestine. Tissue Eng Part A 2018; 24(13–14):1138–47.

134. Rocha FG, Sundback CA, Krebs NJ, et al. The effect of sustained delivery of vascular endothelial growth factor on angiogenesis in tissue-engineered intestine. Biomaterials 2008;29(19):2884–90.

135. Minardi S, Pandolfi L, Taraballi F, et al. Enhancing vascularization through the controlled release of platelet-derived growth factor-BB. ACS Appl Mater Interfaces 2017;9(17):14566–75.

136. Kitano K, Schwartz DM, Zhou H, et al. Bioengineering of functional human induced pluripotent stem cell-derived intestinal grafts. Nat Commun 2017; 8(1). https://doi.org/10.1038/s41467-017-00779-y.

137. Ladd MR, Martin LY, Werts A, et al. The development of newborn porcine models for evaluation of tissue-engineered small intestine. Tissue Eng Part C Methods 2018;24(6):331–45.

138. Schäfer KH, Hagl CI, Rauch U. Differentiation of neurospheres from the enteric nervous system. Pediatr Surg Int 2003;19(5):340–4.

139. Cheng LS, Hotta R, Graham HK, et al. Postnatal human enteric neuronal progenitors can migrate, differentiate, and proliferate in embryonic and postnatal aganglionic gut environments. Pediatr Res 2017;81(5):838–46.

140. Almond S, Lindley RM, Kenny SE, et al. Characterisation and transplantation of enteric nervous system progenitor cells. Gut 2007;56(4):489–96.

141. Lindley RM, Hawcutt DB, Connell MG, et al. Human and mouse enteric nervous system neurosphere transplants regulate the function of aganglionic embryonic distal colon. Gastroenterology 2008;135(1):205–16.e6.

142. Hu H, Ding Y, Mu W, et al. DRG-derived neural progenitors differentiate into functional enteric neurons following transplantation in the postnatal colon. Cell Transplant 2019;28(2):157–69.
143. Workman MJ, Mahe MM, Trisno S, et al. Engineered human pluripotent-stem-cell-derived intestinal tissues with a functional enteric nervous system. Nat Med 2017;23(1):49–59.
144. Schlieve CR, Fowler KL, Thornton M, et al. Neural crest cell implantation restores enteric nervous system function and alters the gastrointestinal transcriptome in human tissue-engineered small intestine. Stem Cell Reports 2017;9(3):883–96.

Bench to Bedside
Approaches for Engineered Intestine, Esophagus, and Colon

Daniel Levin, MD

KEYWORDS

- Tissue engineered intestine • Tissue engineered esophagus
- Tissue engineered colon • Regenerative medicine • Stem cells • Intestinal failure
- Short bowel syndrome

KEY POINTS

- Common approaches to tissue engineering involved isolation of a cell source, preparation of scaffold, and implantation into the host.
- Cell sources are typically pluripotent or multipotent stem cells, the most common being lineage-defined adult stem cells or mesenchymal stems cells.
- The ideal scaffold is biologically inert, absorbable, structurally stable, supportive of cell adherence, inexpensive, and simple to manufacture, store, handle.
- Tissue engineered intestine will eliminate intestinal failure and immunosuppression. Bioengineered esophagus and colon will restore function without sacrificing other organs for gastrointestinal reconstruction.
- Translation to human therapy is nearly available and requires strict adherence to ethical guidelines before introduction.

INTRODUCTION

Management options for patients with intestinal failure have improved dramatically over time. As has been discussed elsewhere in this issue, dietary modification, supplementation, and total parenteral nutrition offer nutritional support for those in need. Among patients with short bowel syndrome, bowel elongation surgery may offer the opportunity to enhance absorptive surface area. For the most severely afflicted and refractory cases, allograft transplantation may offer nutritional autonomy, but comes with several limitations, including lifelong immunosuppression, opportunistic infections, post-transplant lymphoproliferative disease, and a modest 62% 10-year survival.[1] It is these shortcomings that has led some researchers to pursue tissue

Disclosure Statement: None.
Division of Pediatric Surgery, Department of Surgery, University of Virginia, 1300 Jefferson Park Avenue, PO BOX 800709, Charlottesville, VA 22908-0709, USA
E-mail address: Dl2ju@virginia.edu

Gastroenterol Clin N Am 48 (2019) 607–623
https://doi.org/10.1016/j.gtc.2019.08.012
0889-8553/19/© 2019 Elsevier Inc. All rights reserved.

engineered approaches. The ability to harvest one's own cells and subsequently grow a gastrointestinal replacement to fully restore nutritional independence would eliminate the need for harmful immunosuppressive medications. Innovation in the field of bioengineered intestinal replacement is progressing rapidly and translation from bench to bedside is on the horizon. In this article, we aim to put the techniques for tissue engineering in historical perspective, describe common and overlapping concepts, and highlight some of the recent advancements in the development of tissue engineered esophagus, small intestine, and colon.

HISTORY OF GASTROINTESTINAL TISSUE ENGINEERING

- *An abridged history*: Naturally, there are many other important contributions to the field that have not been mentioned in this brief historical perspective of gastrointestinal tissue engineering. Nevertheless, it provides a solid foundation to understand the exciting and fascinating discoveries that are discussed here.
- *1980s—Intestinal cell cultures*: The origins of tissue engineered intestine can be traced back to the 1980s in which early in vitro experiments were designed to optimize intestinal cell cultures.[2]
- *1990s—Establishing tissue engineering techniques*: In the 1990s, Vacanti and colleagues of the Massachusetts General Hospital are credited with the first description of the classic technique currently used to generate tissue engineered small intestine. Namely, they adapted the rat intestinal cellular isolation techniques described by others and used these cells to seed tubularized scaffolds that could then be seeded into host rats for the generation of engineered neointestine.[3]
- *2000s—Tissue engineered intestine can be used to treat short bowel syndrome in animal models*: Grikscheit and colleagues[4] demonstrated that rats with short bowel syndrome could effectively be rescued by anastomosis of tissue engineered constructs in continuity with their native intestine. Subsequently, in 2009, these techniques were applied to a preclinical feasibility study in a Yorkshire swine model.[5]
- *2010s—Human bioengineered intestine is first derived from postnatal tissue*: Researchers at the Children's Hospital Los Angeles isolated cells from pediatric donor tissue and implanted into immunocompromised murine hosts. This marked the first time human small intestine was grown from a nonfetal cell source.[6]
- *Present*: Efforts to improve cell source,[7,8] scaffold,[9,10] neointestinal architecture,[11] and the restoration of the enteric nervous system[12] have been central to many of the recent discoveries and are discussed in greater detail elsewhere in this article.
- *Esophagus and colon engineering*: The history and progress of tissue engineered esophagus and colon has paralleled that of the small intestine. Techniques to generate engineered esophagus began in the 1990s by seeding scaffolds with oral mucosal cells[13] and Nakase and colleagues[14] demonstrated successful replacement of the esophagus in a canine model using tissue engineered esophagus by 2008. Colonic epithelial cultures have been used for decades to study intestinal physiology and colorectal malignancy. A review of these cell lines is beyond the scope of this article. However, in reference to tissue engineered colon specifically as a whole organ colonic replacement, the Vacanti laboratory was successful in translating their early success in tissue engineered small intestine to generate bioengineered colon.[15] Traditionally, efforts to generate tissue

engineered colon have been less enthusiastic. This is largely due to the fact that total proctocolectomy is not life threatening. However, it remains quality of life limiting and engineering efforts have brought about techniques to generate murine bioengineered colon[16] and to repopulate murine and human engineered colon with enteric neurons[17] for the treatment of colonic aganglionosis (Hirschsprung's disease).

COMMON APPROACHES TO TISSUE ENGINEERING

Bioengineering in the alimentary tract involves many overlapping techniques. When distilled down to the most basic concepts, the technique for tissue engineering involves isolation of a cell source, a scaffold mechanism, and host as demonstrated in **Fig. 1**. In many instances, the donor and host is an experimental animal. Many times, the use of experimental animal models is necessary for the research to take place. At all times, the researcher must be in full compliance with the principles of the Institutional Animal Care and Use Committee for the research institute conducting the investigations. The mandates to minimize pain and distress, adequately train personnel, and maintain veterinary oversight must be adhered to. Where possible, the principles of reduction, refinement, and replacement must be considered when designing experiments. In certain instances, for example, a living host may be replaced by bioreactors to generate tissue constructs. This section introduces concepts that are broadly applicable to tissue engineering of all types before moving on to recent advancements in bioengineered esophagus, small intestine, and colon.

Cell Source

- *Ideal cell source:* The preferred cell source contains stem cells; that is, undifferentiated cells capable of self-renewal as well as being able to give rise to multiple cells types through differentiation. In tissue engineering, the stem cell source is preferentially either pluripotent (capable of producing all cells in the body) or multipotent (capable of producing multiple cell types, but not all cell types). The hierarchy of stem cells is demonstrated in **Fig. 2**. Tissue engineered organs derived from both embryonic and adult stem cells have been described.
- *Embryonic stem cells:* It has been more than 2 decades since human embryonic stem cells were derived from blastocysts.[18] These pluripotent cells possess a robust potential to proliferate and differentiate generating fully scalable engineered organs. The numerous therapeutic and biologic discoveries attributable

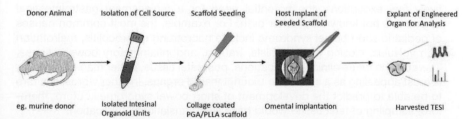

Donor Animal	Isolation of Cell Source	Scaffold Seeding	Host Implant of Seeded Scaffold	Explant of Engineered Organ for Analysis
eg. murine donor	Isolated Intesinal Organoid Units	Collage coated PGA/PLLA scaffold	Omental implantation	Harvested TESI

Fig. 1. The most common steps to experimental tissue engineering. Highlighted are the identification of donor tissue and subsequent isolation of a pluripotent or multipotent cell source. These cells are seeded onto a scaffold and implanted into a host or bioreactor in some instances. After a period of growth, the engineered tissue is harvested for analysis. In the above diagram, the generation of tissue engineered small intestine (TESI) is depicted. PGA, polyglycolic acid; PLLA, poly-ʟ-lactic acid.

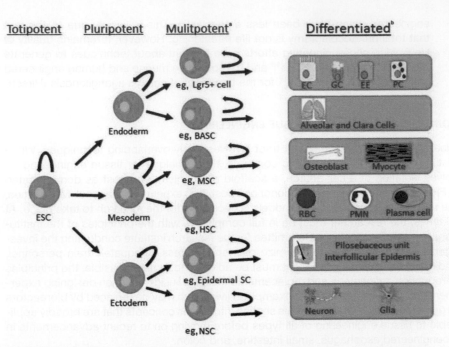

Fig. 2. Simplified schematic of stem cell hierarchy. Totipotent embryonic stem cells (ESCs) are capable of self-renewal and/or give rise to other cells of increasing lineage specificity. Stem cells from the pluripotent germ layers are capable of self-renewal, but are further lineage defined than ESC and capable of generating multipotent cells of increasing tissue specificity. BASC, bronchoalveolar stem cell; EC, enterocyte; EE, enteroendocrine cell; Epidermal SC, epidermal stem cell; GC, goblet cell; HSC, hematopoietic stem cell; Lgr5, leucine-rich repeat-containing G-protein coupled receptor 5; MSC, mesenchymal stem cell; NSC, neural stem cell; PC, Paneth cell; PMN, polymorphonuclear neutrophil; RBC, red blood cell. [a] Simplification. Numerous progenitor cells are not depicted. [b] Simplification. Numerous differentiated cells are not depicted.

to this potential is beyond the scope of this text. As they relate to tissue engineered intestine, this cell source has yielded impressive results.[8] Nevertheless, the potential ethical concerns and controversies over their role in science and medicine has steered many toward alternative cell sources. Moreover, with relatively few exceptions, the potential need for a replacement gastrointestinal segment is not known until after birth. For example, the most common causes of pediatric short bowel syndrome include necrotizing enterocolitis, malrotation with volvulus, closing gastroschisis, trauma, and inflammatory bowel disease. Therefore, in future clinical applications, postnatal tissue, rather than fetal tissue, is most appealing as a source for bioengineered organs. In other words, it is rare to be able to predict the development of short bowel syndrome in utero; therefore, sampling of fetal tissue would have less translational application.[6]

- *Adult stem cells:* For the generation of whole organs, however, pluripotency may not be a requirement. Although adult stem cells, also referred to as somatic stem cells (because these stem cells are found in neonates, children, and adults) are not pluripotent, they maintain multipotency[19–21] and have been an effective cell source for tissue engineered organs.[6] These adult stem cells are lineage restricted to renew and maintain the cells that comprise the organs in which they reside. As an example, the intestinal epithelium is maintained by 2 populations of multipotent cells that are capable of producing additional progenitor cells as well as daughter cells capable of differentiation into all types of mucosal epithelial cells. These cells are either crypt-based columnar cells marked by leucine-rich repeat-containing G-protein coupled receptor 5 or are located at or near position 4 within the intestinal crypts and may be marked by DCAMKL-1 r Bmi-1. Although these cells are capable of producing nearly all cells of the intestinal epithelium, they cannot, for example, produce cardiomyocytes. This limits their usefulness in tissue engineering to the generation of tissue engineered intestine.[22]

- *Mesenchymal stem cells:* The search for additional multipotent cell sources has led some to explore the regenerative potential of mesenchymal stem cells (MSCs). These MSCs represent a broad population of multipotent cells that are derived from mesenchymal and stromal tissues. They are particularly attractive to the field of regenerative medicine because they can be isolated from many adult tissues without difficulty. The earliest research was in MSCs isolated from bone marrow, but additional sources, particularly from amniotic fluid, have sparked a lot of interest for their potential role in immunomodulation, tissue repair, and engineering. Their use in the generation of tissue engineered products is more typically for generation of mesodermal structures such as cartilage, bone, and integument.[23–25] Nevertheless, as it relates to engineering of endodermal structures, such as the esophagus, small intestine and colon, they may still have a role in augmenting the generation of the smooth muscle layers of these organs.[26] Numerous techniques to isolate and purify cellular sources are explored in the literature. Once isolated, these cells are frequently seeded onto a scaffold.

- *Induced pluripotent stem cells*: In efforts to overcome some of the ethical and translational challenges presented by embryonic stem cells while still maintaining the benefit of pluripotency, some have turned to induced pluripotent stem cells. In 2006, Takahashi and Yamanaka[27] described the generation of induced pluripotent stem cells from adult fibroblast cultures via the addition of defined factorsas illustrated in **Fig. 3**. Among many other fascinating applications, induced

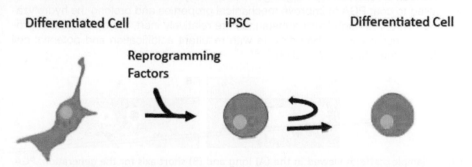

Differentiated Cell   **iPSC**   **Differentiated Cell**

Reprogramming
Factors

eg, Fibroblast

Fig. 3. Simplified schematic of induced pluripotent stem cells (iPSCs). These are derived from differentiated cells, such as fibroblasts, but have also been derived from keratinocytes, renal epithelium, and peripheral blood samples. Induction of transcription factors such as Oct4, Sox2, cMyc and Klf4 can reprogram these cells to a pluripotent state capable of self-renewal and generation of differentiated cells from all germ layers.

pluripotent stem cells have served as effective cell sources for the generation of bioengineered organs.[25,28]

Scaffold

Tissue engineering scaffolds can be categorized into 3 broad categories: synthetic, composite, and biologic.

- *Ideal scaffold:* Characteristics of an ideal scaffold should several properties. The scaffold should be biologically inert; that is, implantation of the material into the host should not illicit an immune reaction or significantly alter the cellular milieu. The scaffold should be absorbable by the host such that the biological tissue will completely replace the synthetic material. This is particularly important in engineering products for pediatric patients, because transplantation of a static material into a growing individual may result in eventual tearing, tugging, mismatch, or erosion at the site of biologic and synthetic interface. The scaffold should possess a structural stability similar to the organ or extracellular matrix (ECM) it seeks to replace. For example, the replacement of bone will have a more firm scaffold material than bowel. The scaffold should be sufficiently porous to allow for cellular imbibition before neovascularization. In addition, the material should be capable of supporting cell adherence, proliferation, and growth and not prevent the clearance of necrotic cells or cellular debris. A product that is stable for storage at room temperature as well as being simple to manufacture, handle, and inexpensive to create is preferred.[29] To date, no single product possess all of these characteristics. Commonly used materials are discussed elsewhere in this article.
- *Synthetic scaffolds:* The most commonly encountered materials are the biodegradable polyglycolic acid (PGA), polycaprolactone, and poly-dl-lactic-co-glycolic acid. These synthetic materials can be woven or electrospun into fabrics with varying density and porosity based on the cell source and host characteristics being used (Examples are demonstrated in **Fig. 4.**). They are hydrolyzed when implanted into a living host and relatively inexpensive. They can be fashioned into different shapes or tubularized, for example, in the generation of conduit or reservoir-type organ generation. Poly-L-lactic acid (PLLA) is frequently used to coat PGA to improve mechanical properties and prolong the hydrolyzation time. Although these substances are relatively inert, the hydrolyzation process does create carbon dioxide with resultant acidification and potential cell loss at the site of implantation.[30,31]

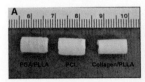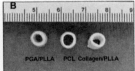

Fig. 4. Sample scaffolds viewed in the (A) long and (B) short axis for the generation. PGA, polyglycolic acid; PCL, polycaprolactone; PLLA, poly-L-lactic acid. (*From* Liu, Y., et al., *Comparison of polyglycolic acid, polycaprolactone, and collagen as scaffolds for the production of tissue engineered intestine.* J Biomed Mater Res B Appl Biomater, 2018; with permission.)

- *Composite scaffolds:* To improve some of the biocompatibility and cell adherence shortcomings of these synthetic materials, some chose to create composite materials by coating or creating them with biologic compounds such as collagen or hyaluronic acid.[31–33] Additional inorganic scaffold materials have included glass, ceramic, and hydroxyapatite.[34] These synthetic and composite scaffolds have improve significantly in recent years.

- *Biologic scaffolds:* Despite advancements in synthetic and composite scaffolds, they do not perfectly recreate the architecture or ECM of native tissue. To improve this structure, some tissue engineers have created biologic scaffolds via whole organ decellularization. The goal is to remove all cells and antigenic determinants and leave behind only the epitope free components of the ECM, such as type 1 collagen, glycosaminoglycans, glycoproteins, and growth factors. These scaffolds maintain the 3-dimensional architecture of the desired organ with the goal to repopulate the organ with donor cells. There is also some evidence that, in addition to structural support, these ECM components may promote cell survival and proliferation.[35]

Host

- *Engineered tissue growth:* Once a suitable scaffold is selected, they can be seeded with isolated or cultured cells and then positioned in an environment to support the growth of the engineered organ. There are 2 predominant environments, namely, living hosts and bioreactors.
- *Living host:* When working with living hosts, one must determine the appropriate experimental model and implantation site. A variety of host animals have been used for the successful generation of tissue engineered organs. Many of the early studies were performed in rats.[4] The introduction of tissue engineering into mice and the numerous transgenic strains available in this animal model offers an opportunity to decipher the genetic mechanisms of tissue engineering.[36] As the technology advances, preclinical studies have necessitated the introduction into larger vertebrate animals such as dogs,[37] sheep,[38,39] pigs,[5,40] and others. Regardless of the experimental model, appropriate matching of the host and donor to avoid graft rejection is important. This process is accomplished by using syngeneic host animals or immunocompromised hosts when the donor and host are of different species.[6] In preclinical and future applications of this technology, however, the donor and host are the same individual, eliminating the risk of rejection.
- *Implantation site:* Within the host animal, the seeded scaffold must be implanted into a favorable location that will support imbibition of nutrients until neovascularization occurs. The most common implantation sites include subcutaneous,[41] renal subcapsular,[42] and omental.[8,15] There are advantages and shortcomings to all of these sites.
  - ○ *Subcutaneous:* The subcutaneous implants are technically less challenging, can easily be harvested, and may be more suitable for the engineering of structures such as bone, cartilage, and muscle. This characteristic is less desirable for intraperitoneal or retroperitoneal structures. For example, if an intestinal segment is grown in the subcutaneous space of the host, to anastomose it in continuity with the native intestine, one would have to harvest it from the subcutaneous space, likely dividing its blood supply, then perform a laparotomy and reestablish vascular inflow and outflow. This vascular anastomosis adds complexity and risk to the case. Therefore, for abdominal viscera, methods that facilitate the development of a vascular pedicle that would not mandate division would eliminate the need for microvascular anastomosis.
  - ○ *Renal capsule:* The renal capsule provides a tight space that allows close apposition of donor tissue and host that may improve graft survival,[43] but is

also retroperitoneal, less mobile, and may compromise renal function in the event of infection or scarring.

o *Omentum:* The omental location offers a well-vascularized, intraperitoneal location with subsequent development of a favorable vascular pedicle.[36] However, the omentum in small vertebrates can be very thin, complicating donor and host apposition and engraftment.

- *Bioreactor:* Generation of engineered organs outside of a living host would offer several advantages, including ex vivo monitoring of the graft development, as well as the ability to precisely control environmental factors (pH, temperature, oxygen content, etc), generate multiple grafts simultaneously, and eliminate any surgical risk that might be imparted during the initial seeded scaffold implantation. In the most basic definition, a bioreactor is a closed device that is capable of supporting conditions that are compatible with cellular differentiation and proliferation. There are many different examples, but there is typically a culture reservoir or chamber containing cells or tissue within a supportive media with inflow and outflow circuits. Flow within the circuit may be passive or supported by a pump. Within the system, delivery of growth factors, inhibitors, additional cell types, and other elements may be perfused. Methods to apply compression, or mechanical or hydrostatic forces are just a few examples of external influences that can be applied. These devices have been used successfully for the growth and manipulation of tissues such as intestine, cartilage, bone, skin, and vascular grafts to name a few,[44,45] but cannot completely reproduce all the biological functions of a living organism. For this reason, although epithelial and stromal cells can be maintained and grown in 3-dimensional cultures, they are, with a few early experimental exceptions, not yet capable of cultivating full-thickness tissue for in vivo transplantation.

TISSUE ENGINEERED INTESTINE

As mentioned, there is a critical need to be able to replace diseased or absent small intestine. Much of the focus in gastrointestinal tissue engineering is on creating strategies for small intestine replacement. Unlike the colon, one cannot live without their small bowel. Unlike the esophagus, one cannot replace it with an imperfect, but survivable, alternative as is the case with gastric or intestinal conduit. This section discusses the current state of the science and focus on recent advancements and concepts in tissue engineered small intestine. The ultimate goal is to be able to grow fully functioning bioengineered intestine that is capable of replacing diseased or absent small bowel. Interestingly, to successfully transition from bench to bedside, however, one does not necessarily need to be able to generate hundreds of centimeters of small bowel. For many patients dependent on total parenteral nutrition, just a few additional centimeters of absorptive surface area could be sufficient to impart clinical benefit and achieve nutritional independence. With this concept in mind, the field is far closer to clinical application in humans than many physicians realize.

- *Engineered neomucosa:* Clearly, the most important function of the small intestine is the absorption of nutrients, minerals and water. For this reason, much attention has been paid to bioengineering of the epithelial lining of the intestine. Current techniques to generate a neomucosa have been quite successful in generating crypts and villi that are nearly indistinguishable from native mucosa on high power magnification.[36] To generate this bioengineered intestine, researchers isolate intestinal organoid units, which are multicellular clusters containing the intestinal epithelial stem cells and their supportive niche cells.

Tubularized PGA/PLLA scaffolds coated in collagen are tubularized, seeded with the organoid units, and implanted into a host animal. This technique and similar techniques have been used by several laboratories to reliably reproduce these results.[4,7,40] A histologic example of tissue engineered small intestine is provided in **Fig. 5**.

- *Differentiated cells of intestinal epithelium are present*: Modern examples of bio-engineered intestine demonstrates all differentiated cells of the intestinal epithelium including enterocytes, enteroendocrine cells, goblet cells, and Paneth cells in normal proportion and distribution.[36]
- *Does tissue engineered intestine function?* There is good evidence to suggest the neomucosa of bioengineered intestine is functional. Tissue engineered intestine demonstrates intact tight junctions, ion channels, and functional glucose transporters and intestinal alkaline phosphatase, all necessary components of a functioning absorptive layer.[46] The epithelial stem cell compartment is intact as well as the periepithelial mesenchymal sheath, including the intestinal subepithelial myofibroblasts.[47,48] However, fully functioning intestine is far more than just an absorptive and secretory epithelial lining and there are several barriers to the clinical translation of the tissue engineered intestine that are active areas of research.
- *Surface area yield remains a barrier to clinical translation:* Currently, the absorptive surface area that can be generated is relatively modest. On average, a 3-fold

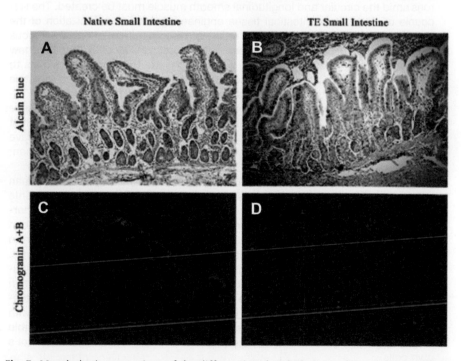

Fig. 5. Morphologic comparison of the differentiated endothelium of the native small intestine and tissue-engineered small intestine. (*A*) and (*B*) Alcian blue staining of goblet cells (original magnification ×10). (*C*) and (*D*) Immunofluorescence staining of enteroendocrine cells using an antichromogranin A+ B primary antibody (original magnification ×40). (*From* Sala, F.G., et al., *Tissue-engineered small intestine and stomach form from autologous tissue in a preclinical large animal model.* J Surg Res, 2009. 156(2): p. 205-12; with permission.)

increase in cell mass can be achieved. For example, if 1 million cells are implanted, the engineered intestine will grow to approximately 3 million cells. In a Lewis rat model, a similar small volume of engineered intestine was sufficient to rescue animals with short bowel syndrome after anastomosis of the engineered segment in continuity with the shortened native intestine. Importantly, the authors showed that, to derive benefit, it was not necessary to restore a normal length of intestine.[4] Nevertheless, improving the surface area yield and size of the bioengineered construct is an important goal. Attempts to enhance and optimize this yield have included overexpression of vascular endothelial growth facgtor,[49] fibroblast growth factor 10 gene,[50] and epidermal growth factor embedded scaffolds.[51] These growth factor enhanced techniques have demonstrated increases in engineered construct size and weight, as well as an increase in the absorptive surface area via deepening of crypts and lengthening of villi. These effects are similar to the beneficial effects of intestinal adaptation and would be expected to improve the absorptive capacity of the engineered intestine.

- Can tissue engineered intestine undergo peristalsis? Beyond the size and length of the engineered intestine, efforts to improve components of the submucosa and muscularis are ongoing. For optimal function, not only must the engineered intestine absorb, it should also undergo peristalsis. To do this, the intricate and interlaced arrangement of the submucosal and myenteric plexus of enteric neurons amid the circular and longitudinal smooth muscle must be created. The first couple of decades of intestinal tissue engineering saw an optimization of the mucosa and it is likely that the next article of bioengineered intestine will focus heavily on these muscle and nerves of the intestine. Recently, exciting new developments on these fronts have been described. Traditional techniques to generate tissue engineered intestine have produced an engineered intestine that lacks a normal enteric nervous system. To overcome this limitation, researchers have been successful in restoring the enteric nervous system of tissue engineered intestine by supplementing the cell source with enteric neural crest cells.[12] Additionally, work to generate contracting sheets of muscularis have demonstrated feasibility for future work to create an intestinal replacement capable of peristalsis.[52]

- When can we expect begin human trials? Researchers have generated human tissue engineered intestine from postnatal pediatric patients. Pediatric patients undergoing intestinal resection for a variety of indications were consented to harvest intestinal organoid units from segments of intestine that would have been otherwise discarded by pathologists. The engineered intestine was grown in an immunocompromised mouse house and subsequently harvested for analysis. This process demonstrated an important proof of concept in the growth of human bioengineered intestine. Nevertheless, it remains difficult to predict when the transition from bench to bedside will take place for tissue engineered intestine. Research in engineered intestine is very active and enthusiastic, and with each new discovery the field inches closer to the eventual goal of being able to generate a fully functional intestinal replacement derived from a patient's own cells.

TISSUE ENGINEERED ESOPHAGUS

The development of tissue engineered esophagus has mirrored the small intestine in many ways. Esophagectomy for cancer, caustic ingestions, and long gap esophageal atresia pose several surgical challenges, such as its location near numerous vital structures and difficult access, relative poor perfusion, an anastomosis prone to tension, and the increased risk associated with anastomotic leak in the mediastinum. The esophagus is more than a simple conduit from mouth to stomach and is, therefore, not amenable to simple interposition with synthetic conduits, as has been attempted in the past. The mucosa, submucosa, muscularis propria, and adventitial layers of the esophagus all serve to participate in the complex esophageal phase of swallowing. Current replacement strategies mandate the sacrifice of other organs, such as the stomach, jejunum, or colon. None of these surgical options is a perfect replacement and are prone to stricture, dilation, stasis, poor function, leak, sepsis, and a host of other complications. Additional strategies, such as gastrostomy tube and esophagostomy deprive the patient of the joys of eating and is associated with an exceptionally poor quality of life. Therefore, a bioengineered esophageal replacement would offer considerable benefit.[53]

- Status of tissue engineered esophagus
  - *Animal models:* The generation of fully engineered intestine is nearing clinical translation. Implantation of collagen coated PGA/PLLA scaffolds seeded with rat derived esophageal progenitor cells and implanted into a rat host can generate a bioengineered esophagus that can be positioned as an interposition graft in the rat. These rats are subsequently able to feed and gain weight.[54] Similar techniques can be performed in mice to gain access to transgenic strains for mechanistic inquiry or human tissue as proof-of-concepts studies.[55] Additional scaffolding sources such as acellular rat esophageal ECM,[56] tubularized acellular porcine bladder ECM,[57] acellular porcine intestinal ECM,[58] and others have demonstrated promise in the generation of esophageal replacement tissue. A model of rat esophageal replacement was recently described wherein the bioengineered esophagus was created from 3-dimensional printed scaffolds seeded with MSC and cultivated in a bioreactor.[59] In 2018, Urbani and colleagues[60] described a multistage and layered technique for the creation of engineered esophagus that seeks to harness the benefits of multiple techniques to generate both the muscular and epithelial layers in a well-vascularized construct. The scaffold is a decellularized rat esophagus. The muscular layer is derived via co-seeding with human mesangioblasts, murine fibroblasts, and murine neural crest cells in a bioreactor cultivation. These cultivated scaffolds were implanted into the omentum of an immunodeficient mouse host. A week later, after neovascularization had begun, the implanted scaffolds were accessed intraoperatively and seeded intraluminally with rat esophageal epithelial cells. Later, the engineered esophagus was harvested and evaluated demonstrating regenerated muscularis externa, submucosa and mucosa, creating one of the most optimized esophageal replacements to date.
  - *Preclinical studies:* As the science progresses, larger mammalian models have demonstrated important preclinical feasibility. Catry and colleagues[61] have demonstrated the survival of pigs after 3-cm-long full-thickness esophageal replacement with tissue engineered esophagus. They have demonstrated an acceleration of the reepithelization of their engineered constructs via utilization of MSC-seeded matrices. Similarly, La Francesca and colleagues[62] have demonstrated successful porcine esophageal engineering with retrievable synthetic stents seeded with MSCs. Before translation in human, however, additional work to predict long term outcomes and function will need to be done.

○ *Application of similar technology in the treatment of human disease:* Although a fully functional engineered esophagus has yet to be implanted in humans, esophageal repair via regenerative medicine techniques has made the transition to human therapy. In 2011, Badylak and colleagues[63] described their technique for endoscopic esophageal mucosectomy for Barrett's esophagus with high-grade dysplasia followed by endoluminal lining of the resection field with a xenogeneic ECM. All patients healed with minimal stricture and complete replacement of the ECM by squamous epithelium. Using techniques similar to tissue engineering, Dua and colleagues[64] describe the successful repair of a 5-cm traumatic esophageal injury in a 24-year-old man that was not amenable to more traditional repair or temporizing techniques. They were able to repair the full-thickness gap with an endoluminal esophageal stent that was subsequently externally covered, via open cervical incision, by a commercially available acellular dermal matrix coated in the patient's own platelet-rich plasma. Four years after stent removal, the patient is doing well, taking all nutrition by mouth.[64] Although it is not a fully engineered esophagus, this notable accomplishment underscores the potential impact of this technology, and others like it, in the treatment of human disease. The authors obtained approval to implement this technology under compassionate grounds. The success in this patient should not prompt immediate human translation without further study, because this technology does not yet represent a change in the recommended management of these types of esophageal injuries. This example underscores the importance of continued research before widespread translation in humans. The application of tissue engineered organ replacement in humans should not be undertaken until it is fully understood and patients can be properly informed.

TISSUE ENGINEERED COLON

As stated, colonic epithelial cell lines have been used for decades to investigate colorectal carcinoma, inflammatory bowel disease, and infectious colitis. However, the sizable interest in colonic cell lines is not met by an equal interest in generating full-thickness colonic replacement. This is due in large part to the fact that total colectomy is survivable without a replacement and, in many patients, an ileostomy can be avoided or closed via ileoanal or ileal pouch anastomosis. The small bowel is capable of absorbing all water that is needed to survive and will adapt to mitigate the lost volume of absorption that takes place during colonic dehydration of stool. Additionally, concentrations of sodium, magnesium, and bile acids, for example, can be maintained within the normal limit despite loss of colonic absorption. Similarly, dietary intake of vitamin K and biotin is typically sufficient to avoid deficiency in those vitamins produced by probiotic bacteria. Nevertheless, loss of the colon drastically increases the frequency of stooling, which can increase the risk of dehydration or electrolyte derangement if oral intake is insufficient or in times of acute gastrointestinal illness. These factors can lead to a decrease in quality of life that could be obviated by an engineered colonic replacement.

• *Advancements in colon engineering parallel small intestine:* As one would anticipate, the early success in the generation of tissue engineered small intestine was replicated with colonic tissue. The creation of colonic organoid units seeded on a collagen coated PGA/PLLA scaffold and implanted into the omentum of host rats will generate a colonic construct that is histologically similar to native colon. When anastomosed in gastrointestinal continuity of the experimental animal, this group of rats lost less body weight, had increased intestinal transit time, increased dry stool weight, and increased serum bile acid and short chain fatty acid concentration in comparison to control groups without engineered colon.[15] The future success of tissue engineered colon is encouraged by the fact that human tissue will grow in an immunocompromised mouse host.[16]

- *Tissue engineered colon as a model to study colon physiology and disease:* In addition to the goal of developing engineered colon as large intestine replacement, seeded scaffold techniques have demonstrated usefulness in 3-dimensional models of colonic drug delivery to investigate treatments for in-flammatory bowel disease[65] and to mimic colon cancer metastasis.[66] Moreover, overlapping technologies may someday be used to repopulate aganglionic colon with enteric neurons and glia to cure enteric neuropathies.[17,67] Overall, current studies suggest that, as the experience in tissue engineered small intestine grows, these lessons and engineering strategies can be successfully applied to colon such that bench to bedside translation is likely to keep pace with bio-engineered small bowel.

FUTURE DIRECTIONS AND ETHICAL CONSIDERATIONS

Regarding tissue engineered small intestine, the field has seen dramatic improve-ments in the purification of cell sources, creation of scaffold materials, and generation of intact neomucosa. The future will see research aimed at overcoming many of the current limitations. Most striking among these current limitations are the volume of engineered intestine and the mesodermal derived components of the intestine. Enhancing these will permit replacement of large segments of small intestine that is replete with an organized muscularis, enteric nervous system and lymphatic system. Additionally, parallel research into humanization of xenografts and/or induced immu-notolerance may make organ replacement via xenograft a viable option in the future.

The application of stem cell biology in tissue engineering must be performed with thought and dignity. The tissue engineer must embrace the pluripotent character of stem cells to create organs, while not crossing internationally accepted norms and bans on human cloning. Introduction into human therapy can only be considered when the safety of the technology has been clearly demonstrated in experimental models and subjects are well informed. Moving too quickly creates unacceptable risk to human subjects and patients.[68] As refinement and optimization of tissue engi-neering methods improve, a greater emphasis on human translation is inevitable.

REFERENCES

1. Celik N, Stanley K, Rudolph J, et al. Improvements in intestine transplantation. Semin Pediatr Surg 2018;27:267–72.
2. Evans GS, Flint N, Somers AS, et al. The development of a method for the prep-aration of rat intestinal epithelial cell primary cultures. J Cell Sci 1992;101(Pt 1): 219–31.
3. Choi RS, Vacanti JP. Preliminary studies of tissue-engineered intestine using iso-lated epithelial organoid units on tubular synthetic biodegradable scaffolds. Transpl Proc 1997;29:848–51.
4. Grikscheit TC, Siddique A, Ochoa ER, et al. Tissue-engineered small intestine im-proves recovery after massive small bowel resection. Ann Surg 2004;240:748–54.
5. Sala FG, Kunisaki SM, Ochoa ER, et al. Tissue-engineered small intestine and stomach form from autologous tissue in a preclinical large animal model. J Surg Res 2009;156:205–12.

6. Levin DE, Barthel ER, Speer AL, et al. Human tissue-engineered small intestine forms from postnatal progenitor cells. J Pediatr Surg 2013;48:129–37.
7. Cromeens BP, Liu Y, Stathopoulos J, et al. Production of tissue-engineered intestine from expanded enteroids. J Surg Res 2016;204:164–75.
8. Finkbeiner SR, Freeman JJ, Wieck MM, et al. Generation of tissue-engineered small intestine using embryonic stem cell-derived human intestinal organoids. Biol Open 2015;4:1462–72.
9. Davis LM, Callanan A, Carroll GT, et al. On the potential of hydrated storage for naturally derived ECMs and associated effects on mechanical and cellular performance. J Biomed Mater Res B Appl Biomater 2014;102:89–97.
10. Ladd MR, Costello C, Gosztyla C, et al. Development of intestinal scaffolds that mimic native mammalian intestinal tissue. Tissue Eng A 2019.
11. Liu Y, Rager T, Johnson J, et al. Enriched intestinal stem cell seeding improves the architecture of tissue-engineered intestine. Tissue Eng C Methods 2015;21: 816–24.
12. Schlieve CR, Fowler KL, Thornton M, et al. Neural crest cell implantation restores enteric nervous system function and alters the gastrointestinal transcriptome in human tissue-engineered small intestine. Stem Cell Rep 2017;9:883–96.
13. Natsume T, Ike O, Okada T, et al. Experimental studies of a hybrid artificial esophagus combined with autologous mucosal cells. ASAIO Trans 1990;36:M435–7.
14. Nakase Y, Nakamura T, Kin S, et al. Intrathoracic esophageal replacement by in situ tissue-engineered esophagus. J Thorac Cardiovasc Surg 2008;136:850–9.
15. Grikscheit TC, Ogilvie JB, Ochoa ER, et al. Tissue-engineered colon exhibits function in vivo. Surgery 2002;132:200–4.
16. Barthel ER, Levin DE, Speer AL, et al. Human tissue-engineered colon forms from postnatal progenitor cells: an in vivo murine model. Regen Med 2012;7:807–18.
17. Wieck MM, El-Nachef WN, Hou X, et al. Human and murine tissue-engineered colon exhibit diverse neuronal subtypes and can be populated by enteric nervous system progenitor cells when donor colon is aganglionic. Tissue Eng Part A 2016; 22:53–64.
18. Thomson JA, Itskovitz-Eldor J, Shapiro SS, et al. Embryonic stem cell lines derived from human blastocysts. Science 1998;282:1145–7.
19. Gage FH. Mammalian neural stem cells. Science 2000;287(5457):1433–8.
20. Reynolds BA, Weiss S. Generation of neurons and astrocytes from isolated cells of the adult mammalian central nervous system. Science 1992;255(5052): 1707–10.
21. Toma JG, Akhavan M, Fernandes KJ, et al. Isolation of multipotent adult stem cells from the dermis of mammalian skin. Nat Cell Biol 2001;3:778–84.
22. Umar S. Intestinal stem cells. Curr Gastroenterol Rep 2010;12(5):340–8.
23. Li H, Shen S, Fu H, et al. Immunomodulatory functions of mesenchymal stem cells in tissue engineering. Stem Cells Int 2019;2019:9671206.
24. Marion NW, Mao JJ. Mesenchymal stem cells and tissue engineering. Methods Enzymol 2006;420:339–61.
25. Tang M, Chen W, Liu J, et al. Human induced pluripotent stem cell-derived mesenchymal stem cell seeding on calcium phosphate scaffold for bone regeneration. Tissue Eng Part A 2014;20:1295–305.
26. Hori Y, Nakamura T, Kimura D, et al. Experimental study on tissue engineering of the small intestine by mesenchymal stem cell seeding. J Surg Res 2002;102: 156–60.
27. Takahashi K, Yamanaka S. Induction of pluripotent stem cells from mouse embryonic and adult fibroblast cultures by defined factors. Cell 2006;126(4):663–76.

28. Lin W, Chen M, Hu C, et al. Endowing iPSC-Derived MSCs with Angiogenic and Keratinogenic differentiation potential: a promising cell source for skin tissue engineering. Biomed Res Int 2018;2018:8459503.
29. Patel M, Fisher JP. Biomaterial scaffolds in pediatric tissue engineering. Pediatr Res 2008;63(5):497–501.
30. O'Brien FJ. Biomaterials & Scaffolds for tissue engineering. Mater Today 2011; 14(3):88–95.
31. Liu Y, Nelson T, Chakroff J, et al. Comparison of polyglycolic acid, polycaprolactone, and collagen as scaffolds for the production of tissue engineered intestine. J Biomed Mater Res B Appl Biomater 2018.
32. Chircov C, Grumezescu AM, Bejenaru LE. Hyaluronic acid-based scaffolds for tissue engineering. Rom J Morphol Embryol 2018;59(1):71–6.
33. Hemshekhar M, Thushara RM, Chandranayaka S, et al. Emerging roles of hyaluronic acid bioscaffolds in tissue engineering and regenerative medicine. Int J Biol Macromol 2016;86:917–28.
34. Dinarvand P, Seyedjafari E, Shafiee A, et al. New approach to bone tissue engineering: simultaneous application of hydroxyapatite and bioactive glass coated on a poly(L-lactic acid) scaffold. ACS Appl Mater Interfaces 2011;3(11):4518–24.
35. Badylak SF, Taylor D, Uygun K. Whole-organ tissue engineering: decellularization and recellularization of three-dimensional matrix scaffolds. Annu Rev Biomed Eng 2011;13:27–53.
36. Sala FG, Matthews JA, Speer AL, et al. A multicellular approach forms a significant amount of tissue-engineered small intestine in the mouse. Tissue Eng Part A 2011;17(13–14):1841–50.
37. Hiwatashi S, Nakayama Y, Umeda S, et al. Tracheal replacement using an in-body tissue-engineered collagenous tube "BIOTUBE" with a biodegradable stent in a beagle model: a preliminary report on a new technique. Eur J Pediatr Surg 2019;29(1):90–6.
38. Ahmad Z, Al-Wattar Z, Rushton N. Tissue engineering for the ovine rotator cuff: surgical anatomy, approach, implantation and histology technique, along with review of literature. J Invest Surg 2018;1–12.
39. Best CA, Pepper VK, Ohst D, et al. Designing a tissue-engineered tracheal scaffold for preclinical evaluation. Int J Pediatr Otorhinolaryngol 2018;104:155–60.
40. Ladd MR, Martin LY, Werts A, et al. The development of newborn porcine models for evaluation of tissue-engineered small intestine. Tissue Eng Part C Methods 2018;24(6):331–45.
41. Khorramirouz R, Go JL, Noble C, et al. A novel surgical technique for a rat subcutaneous implantation of a tissue engineered scaffold. Acta Histochem 2018; 120(3):282–91.
42. Watson CL, Mahe MM, Múnera J, et al. An in vivo model of human small intestine using pluripotent stem cells. Nat Med 2014;20(11):1310–4.
43. Ohashi K, Tatsumi K, Utoh R, et al. Engineering liver tissues under the kidney capsule site provides therapeutic effects to hemophilia B mice. Cell Transplant 2010;19(6):807–13.
44. Zhao J, Micholle G, Cai J, et al. Bioreactors for tissue engineering; An update. Biochem Eng J 2016;103:268–81.
45. Zhou W, Chen Y, Roh T, et al. Multifunctional bioreactor system for human intestine tissues. ACS Biomater Sci Eng 2018;4(1):231–9.
46. Grant CN, Mojica SG, Sala FG, et al. Human and mouse tissue-engineered small intestine both demonstrate digestive and absorptive function. Am J Physiol Gastrointest Liver Physiol 2015;308(8):G664–77.

47. Worthley DL, Churchill M, Compton JT, et al. Gremlin 1 identifies a skeletal stem cell with bone, cartilage, and reticular stromal potential. Cell 2015;160(1–2): 269–84.

48. Cromeens BP, Wang Y, Liu Y, et al. Critical intestinal cells originate from the host in enteroid-derived tissue-engineered intestine. J Surg Res 2018;223:155–64.

49. Matthews JA, Sala FG, Speer AL, et al. VEGF optimizes the formation of tissue-engineered small intestine. Regen Med 2011;6(5):559–67.

50. Torashima Y, Levin DE, Barthel ER, et al. Fgf10 overexpression enhances the formation of tissue-engineered small intestine. J Tissue Eng Regen Med 2016;10(2): 132–9.

51. Liu Y, Nelson T, Cromeens B, et al. HB-EGF embedded in PGA/PLLA scaffolds via subcritical CO2 augments the production of tissue engineered intestine. Biomaterials 2016;103:150–9.

52. Wang Q, Wang K, Solorzano-Vargas RS, et al. Bioengineered intestinal muscularis complexes with long-term spontaneous and periodic contractions. PLoS One 2018;13(5):e0195315.

53. Arakelian L, Kanai N, Dua K, et al. Esophageal tissue engineering: from bench to bedside. Ann N Y Acad Sci 2018;1434(1):156–63.

54. Grikscheit T, Ochoa ER, Srinivasan A, et al. Tissue-engineered esophagus: experimental substitution by onlay patch or interposition. J Thorac Cardiovasc Surg 2003;126(2):537–44.

55. Spurrier RG, Speer AL, Hou X, et al. Murine and human tissue-engineered esophagus form from sufficient stem/progenitor cells and do not require microdesigned biomaterials. Tissue Eng Part A 2015;21(5–6):906–15.

56. Bhrany AD, Beckstead BL, Lang TC, et al. Development of an esophagus acellular matrix tissue scaffold. Tissue Eng 2006;12(2):319–30.

57. Badylak SF, Vorp DA, Spievack AR, et al. Esophageal reconstruction with ECM and muscle tissue in a dog model. J Surg Res 2005;128(1):87–97.

58. Lopes MF, Cabrita A, Ilharco J, et al. Esophageal replacement in rat using porcine intestinal submucosa as a patch or a tube-shaped graft. Dis Esophagus 2006;19(4):254–9.

59. Kim IG, Wu Y, Park SA, et al. Tissue-engineered esophagus via bioreactor cultivation for circumferential esophageal reconstruction. Tissue Eng Part A 2019. [Epub ahead of print].

60. Urbani L, Camilli C, Phylactopoulos DE, et al. Multi-stage bioengineering of a layered oesophagus with in vitro expanded muscle and epithelial adult progenitors. Nat Commun 2018;9(1):4286.

61. Catry J, Luong-Nguyen M, Arakelian L, et al. Circumferential esophageal replacement by a tissue-engineered substitute using mesenchymal stem cells: an experimental study in mini pigs. Cell Transplant 2017;26(12):1831–9.

62. La Francesca S, Aho JM, Barron MR, et al. Long-term regeneration and remodeling of the pig esophagus after circumferential resection using a retrievable synthetic scaffold carrying autologous cells. Sci Rep 2018;8(1):4123.

63. Badylak SF, Hoppo T, Nieponice A, et al. Esophageal preservation in five male patients after endoscopic inner-layer circumferential resection in the setting of superficial cancer: a regenerative medicine approach with a biologic scaffold. Tissue Eng Part A 2011;17(11–12):1643–50.

64. Dua KS, Hogan WJ, Aadam AA, et al. In-vivo oesophageal regeneration in a human being by use of a non-biological scaffold and extracellular matrix. Lancet 2016;388(10039):55–61.

65. Huang Z, Wang Z, Long S, et al. A 3-D artificial colon tissue mimic for the evaluation of nanoparticle-based drug delivery system. Mol Pharm 2014;11(7): 2051–61.
66. Nietzer S, Baur F, Sieber S, et al. Mimicking metastases including tumor stroma: a new technique to generate a three-dimensional colorectal cancer model based on a biological decellularized intestinal scaffold. Tissue Eng Part C Methods 2016;22(7):621–35.
67. Almond S, Lindley RM, Kenny SE, et al. Characterisation and transplantation of enteric nervous system progenitor cells. Gut 2007;56(4):489–96.
68. Abbott A. Medical Nobel prize committee deals with surgical scandal. Nature 2016;537(7620):289–90.

The Oley Foundation and Consumer Support Groups

Julie M. Andolina, Lisa Crosby Metzger, BA, Joan Bishop*

KEYWORDS

- The Oley Foundation • Support groups • Intestinal failure • Parenteral nutrition
- Enteral nutrition • Home nutrition support • HPN • HEN

KEY POINTS

- Because of the complexity of home parenteral and enteral nutrition (HPEN) therapy and treatment of intestinal failure (IF), HPEN consumers often face depression, isolation, fatigue, anxiety, financial stress, and so on, in addition to the physical effects of IF and HPEN. These stressors affect the families of HPEN consumers as well as the consumers (patients) themselves.
- Research shows HPEN consumers benefit in many ways from participating in Oley Foundation programs.
- Other organizations also offer support, programs, and educational opportunities for HPEN consumers and IF patients.

INTRODUCTION

When someone is diagnosed with a life-altering illness or condition, there is an unmistakable hierarchy assigned to the resulting problems and changes. At first, life for the patient and their family is all about survival and recovery. Time, money, and sometimes comfort are thrown to the wind to ensure that the patient will live to see another day. Family dynamics change; hospital visits take priority over work, school, hobbies, and sometimes other family members. Survival is the top priority. When it comes to chronic illnesses, however, what happens when survival is not a pressing question?

When a chronic medical condition is no longer an imminent threat to the patient's life, everyone feels, of course, a moment of overwhelming relief. However, as time goes on, that relief fades and is replaced by anxiety and uncertainty about the future as the patient and their loved ones learn to manage the condition and the changes it has wrought in their lives. Suddenly, the patient is asked to thrive when he or she has been focused on merely surviving.

Disclosure: Authors are all Oley Foundation staff.
The Oley Foundation, Albany Medical Center, MC 28, 99 Delaware Avenue, Delmar, NY 12054, USA
* Corresponding author.
E-mail address: bishopj@amc.edu

As someone who suffers from short bowel syndrome resulting from a congenital diaphragmatic hernia, I (Julie) am in a unique position to comment on the physical as well as the psychological effects of intestinal failure and the use of home nutrition support.

INTESTINAL FAILURE AND MANAGEMENT

Looking at data it had collected, in 2016 the European Society for Clinical Nutrition and Metabolism (ESPEN) ruled intestinal failure (IF) the rarest form of organ failure.[1] ESPEN defines IF as "the reduction of gut function below the minimum necessary for the absorption of macronutrients and/or water and electrolytes, such that intravenous supplementation is required to maintain health and/or growth." IF may occur suddenly and abruptly (eg, as the result of an accident), or it "may be the slow, progressive evolution of a chronic illness." It may be short term or long lasting (chronic intestinal failure).[2]

Common treatments for IF include parenteral nutrition (PN) and enteral nutrition (EN), often administered long term and at home (HPN and HEN).[3,4] The use of these life-saving treatments comes with many complications, such as the threat of infection, intolerance, and metabolic deviations. Both IF and HPEN come with the often less well-considered or acknowledged psychosocial effects of depression, isolation, fatigue, anxiety, loss of independence, and reliance on technology and caregivers, the inability to eat, interference with friendly, romantic, and sexual relationships, and, in many cases, severe financial stress.[3,5,6]

The source of the IF, whether it is sudden onset or the progressive evolution of a chronic illness; the chosen treatment options, including nutrition support, medical or surgical options; the ongoing effects of the IF, including pain, diarrhea, food intolerance; family support; support of a knowledgeable medical team, or a lack thereof; and other factors, have tremendous effect on how well a patient is able to manage their IF.

PREVALENCE OF HOME PARENTERAL NUTRITION AND HOME ENTERAL NUTRITION

Based on a review of Medicare beneficiary data for 2013 and data provided by 3 of the largest home infusion providers in the United States, Mundi and colleagues[4] estimate that in 2013, 25,011 US inhabitants were sustaining themselves on HPN and 437,882 were dependent on HEN. Of the 25,011 HPN users, approximately 83% were adults, and 17% were pediatric. Comparatively, of the estimated 437,882 HEN users, 57% were adults and 43% were pediatric.

This study was compared with a similar one conducted in 1992 by Howard and colleagues[7] in which the number of HPN and HEN consumers was estimated to be approximately 40,000 and 152,000, respectively. In the 21 years between these studies, the prevalence of HPN has actually decreased, whereas the prevalence of HEN has increased (**Fig. 1**). (A note on terminology: Over the years, Oley Foundation members have expressed a preference for the term "consumer" over "patient." They acknowledge they are "patients" when they are in the hospital, but when they are home, living their lives on HPEN, they prefer to be called "consumers." This term is used from here on.)

When compared with the total population of the United States, these are not large numbers, amounting to 21 Medicare HPN consumers per 1 million US inhabitants and 361 Medicare HEN consumers per million.[4] It is uncommon for a person on HEN or HPN, especially, to know of anyone else on the therapy, and a sense of isolation prevails in this population (**Fig. 2**).

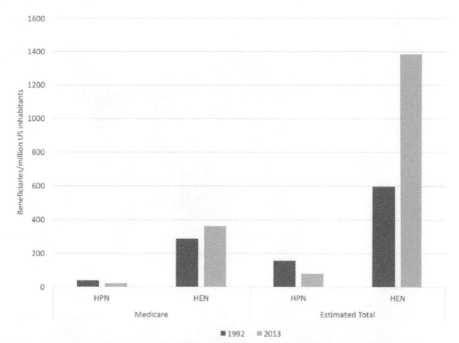

Fig. 1. Prevalence of HPN and HEN for Medicare and estimated total beneficiaries per million US inhabitants for 1992 and 2013. (*From* Mundi MS, Pattinson A, McMahon MT et al. Prevalence of home parenteral and enteral nutrition in the United States. Nutrition in Clinical Practice 2017 Dec;32(6):802; with permission.)

THE EFFECT OF SUPPORT GROUPS ON HOME PARENTERAL NUTRITION AND HOME ENTERAL NUTRITION CONSUMERS

Merriam-Webster defines "support group" as "a group of people with common experiences and concerns who provide emotional and moral support for one another."[8] Metzger and colleagues[6] note that support groups give people "opportunities to talk to others who share a common experience; give and receive emotional support; share problems, concerns, and coping skills; and gather information and learn." Studies have shown that participating in support groups can positively affect patient outcomes in multiple areas for those who suffer from chronic illnesses.[9] There are many different types of health-related support groups in the United States, varying in size, professionalism, meeting regularity, and form of interaction (face to face, over the phone, over video, and so on).[3,6]

Support groups allow people the chance to learn by sharing experiences, problems, concerns, coping skills, and valuable information that can reduce the feeling of isolation or "otherness."[6] In 2002, Carol Smith and others[10] conducted a study to determine how association with the Oley Foundation affected HPN consumers. They concluded that patients affiliated with this support organization had a higher quality of life, less reactive depression, and fewer encounters with catheter-related sepsis than patients who were not affiliated with the organization.

THE OLEY FOUNDATION: MISSION AND HISTORY

The Oley Foundation is a national, independent, not-for-profit organization located in Albany, New York.[11] It is one of several nonprofit organizations that offers support to

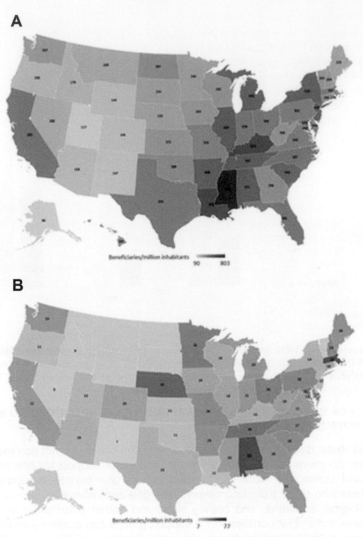

Fig. 2. Number of Medicare beneficiaries per million inhabitants per state for (*A*) HEN and (*B*) HPN. States in gray did not have information available. (*From* Mundi MS, Pattinson A, McMahon MT et al. Prevalence of home parenteral and enteral nutrition in the United States. Nutrition in Clinical Practice 2017 Dec;32(6):803; with permission.)

people with IF and/or on HPEN (see others listed later). The Oley Foundation was founded in 1983 by then Director of the Clinical Nutrition HPEN program at Albany Medical Center in Albany, New York, Dr Lyn Howard, and her long-time patient Clarence "Oley" Oldenburg, and the mission of the Oley Foundation is "to enrich the lives of those living on home intravenous nutrition and tube feeding through education, advocacy, and networking" (Dahl R, Oley Foundation FY 2018 and FY Q1 2019 reports, unpublished).[6]

In 1975, when he was 46 years old, Clarence suffered intestinal ischemia that cut off blood circulation to his intestines. He spent 5 years in the hospital, where he underwent several emergency surgeries and eventually lost most of his small intestine.

He started to get his life back in the early 1980s, when he was referred to Dr Howard at Albany Medical Center, who discharged him on HPN. Dr Howard arranged for her patients who were on HPN, including Clarence, to meet in both formal and informal settings, such as at clinic and at picnics. After realizing how Clarence's quality of life had improved on HPN, and how little was understood about this as an option for home use, his brother, Bill, provided the seed money to get the Oley Foundation started.[12]

Five years before the founding of the Oley Foundation, Lee Koonin, a new HPN user, and her husband, Marshall, started the Lifeline Foundation: a support group for HPN users in Sharon, Massachusetts, striving to reduce feelings of isolation and spread knowledge of the life-saving therapy. In 1977, when Lee was put on HPN, it was still an experimental therapy that was not being used in many hospitals. Lee felt very alone and became determined to connect with others in a similar position. Together, Lee and Marshall published a newsletter, organized picnics, and brought together a network of consumers who were willing to share their knowledge and experiences with other people on HPN. By 1984, the Lifeline Foundation had acquired about 600 members, and it had begun to put a strain on the Koonins in terms of both time and money. After confirming the commitment and dedication of the newly created Oley Foundation, Lee and Marshall put their Lifeline Foundation into the hands of the Oley Foundation staff, giving thanks to Clarence and Dr Howard.[12]

Today, the Oley Foundation continues to provide education, advocacy, and support to its now 21,975 members, made up of HPEN consumers, family members, clinicians, and members of industry.

THE OLEY FOUNDATION: A TYPICAL SUPPORT GROUP?

The Oley Foundation is often referred to as a support group, but it goes well above and beyond that label. In a study of the value of membership in the Oley Foundation to HPN- and/or HEN-dependent people, there arose 4 main themes that membership with Oley provided: competency, inspiration, normalcy, and advocacy[5] (**Fig. 3**).

Competency

Consumers involved in the study stated that they felt more competent in managing their lives on HPEN when they received education and materials from Oley. Because the foundation is made up of consumers and clinicians, new members are able to receive information based on years of personal experience that their specialist or primary care physician may not be able to provide.[5] One mother of an HPEN-dependent child attended an Oley conference and claims to have learned information that saved her son's life. After having his first central line placed at age 3 because of short bowel syndrome that resulted from an intestinal infarction, the woman explains how her son suffered from continuous fevers, a sign of infection, and was in and out of the hospital for 4 months.

In the midst of yet another hospitalization due to a bacterial line infection, this mother took the opportunity to attend the annual Oley conference, which happened to be going on locally. She gathered family and friends to attend and help her learn as much as possible:

"On the first day we split up to cover as many presentations as possible. Later we met in 'headquarters' upstairs in the hotel room, and everybody starts looking at each other saying, 'You know what? You can live on HPN. Our doctor and nurses said you die on HPN! They said he'd never eat. He can eat. You know what? We're not being sterile with the line, and you're not supposed to have a cap with lipid crud coming out the top.'"[6]

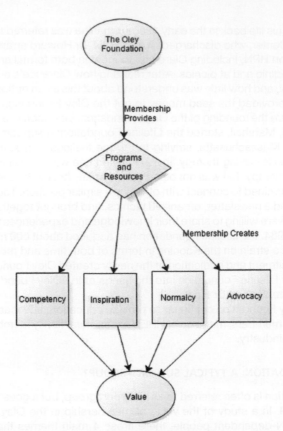

Fig. 3. A conceptual model of value of membership in the Oley Foundation. (*From* Chopy K, Winkler M, Schwartz-Barcott, D et al. A qualitative study of perceived value of membership in the Oley Foundation by home parenteral and enteral nutrition consumers. Journal of Parenteral and Enteral Nutrition 2015 May;39(4):431; with permission.)

Because of the information she received at the conference, this woman's son was not only able to survive, but thrive on HPN, going from spending 70 days of the first 7 months in the hospital, to a total of 7 in-patient days in 8 years. She concludes, "The Oley conference saved his life, there is no question."[6]

Inspiration

Both HPN- and HEN-dependent participants in this study felt a sense of inspiration from being connected to the members of Oley. They expressed that "seeing other people living their life" despite using these therapies was encouraging and helped them to accept their own need for HPN and/or HEN. After seeing images of children living their lives with feeding tubes, backpacks, and pumps, one man said, "[S]urely a grown man who was in the army could tackle it too."[5]

From listening to the stories of others, many participants who had previously viewed their dependence on HPN or HEN as life ending conceded that it was actually a means for people of all ages to "carry on a decent life as long as their disability allows."[5]

Normalcy

By being a part of Oley, consumers felt that they were a part of a community of HPN and HEN users, which significantly decreased feelings of isolation. Participants made note of the strong support system, and the opportunity to see other people with similar conditions thriving in their everyday lives. Contrary to the common assumption, many people affiliated with Oley stated that they felt they could live a completely normal life with their feeding tubes and central lines.[5]

Advocacy

On the topic of advocacy, participants in this study made note of 2 distinct types: the Oley Foundation advocating for HPEN consumers and membership with Oley generating a desire to self-advocate. In regard to the former, participants reported feeling that Oley was there and standing up for consumers; regarding the latter, stories were told of consumers who took it upon themselves to lobby and write letters to congressional leaders, arguing for expanding health care coverage to include HPEN supplies and additives.[5]

OLEY PROGRAMS AND SERVICES

The Oley Foundation provides several valuable programs and services to its members.

Newsletter

Oley publishes 6 bimonthly newsletters a year that are received by approximately 17,000 HPEN consumers, home care providers, and health care professionals in a total of 49 countries. The newsletter, called the *LifelineLetter*, a homage to the Koonins' support group, is published both electronically and physically and includes a wide range of information for consumers. Articles are peer reviewed. Newsletter readers praise its connectivity and valued information. One HPEN consumer said "I LOVE, LOVE, LOVE getting the newsletter. It makes me feel connected, and not so alone!"[13]

Dr Darlene Kelly, Oley's Advisor for Science and Medicine, referring to 1 article published in the *LifelineLetter*, said, "[The article] gives pointers on how patient/consumers and others should critically read healthcare-related websites. It is important to consider the source by observing the address: if it ends in .org, it is a not-for-profit organization, while .gov comes from the government, .edu is from an education/academic institution, and .com is a commercial company. The HONcode, sponsored by the Health on the Network Foundation, is an additional assurance that the not-for-profit websites have continual oversight to assure that they provide trustworthy medical information."[11]

I, myself, have gotten a lot of use out of the *LifelineLetter*, reading the stories of other HPEN consumers during times when I felt abnormal or uncomfortable with my condition. The newsletter certainly does provide a sense of connection and reassurance that you are not alone.

Conferences

At Oley national and regional conferences, HPEN consumers, their families, clinicians, Oley sponsors, and volunteers come together to share research and experiences. In a discussion about Oley, the executive director, Joan Bishop, said about the conferences, "There are education sessions, which are presented by well-known clinicians from the US, Canada, and on occasion from abroad. Breakout sessions give attendees an opportunity to ask questions and to learn more about specific topics. Exhibits introduce attendees to new technology and there are opportunities for networking among those who are on these therapies. Friendships develop, and many become lifelong."[11]

In 2018 to 2019, regional conferences were held in Massachusetts, Ohio, Texas, California, Florida, and Nevada (Dahl R, Oley Foundation FY 2018 and FY Q1 2019 reports, unpublished).

Oley's 2019 annual national conference took place in Chicago, Illinois. It was a collaborative effort with the University of Illinois at Chicago, with exciting presentations and an opportunity for clinicians to earn continuing education credits. A recording of the presentations is available on Oley YouTube channel.

I (Julie) attended for the first time since I was a child. Meeting other HPEN consumers and networking with the faculty gave me a new outlook on my life as a consumer.

Webinars

This online source of education is provided free of charge to everyone. Recorded and later available on Oley's YouTube channel, the Webinars can be viewed by consumers, caregivers, family members, and clinicians in the comfort of their own home.[10] The Webinars cover a wide range of topics, from new technology to coping strategies, and are presented by both clinicians and consumers alike.[14]

Oley Web Site and Information Clearinghouse

Oley responds to hundreds of queries from patients and family members each year, including direct requests for information about managing IF, clogged or leaking tubes, finding a nutrition support clinician, and much more. In fiscal year 2018 (October 1, 2017–September 31, 2018), they had 619,000 page views on the Oley Web site. Resources on the Web site (some also available in print) include complication charts for HEN and HPN (HPN currently under revision); a glossary; links to meet other patients and inspiring patient stories; tips for daily living, such as travel, swimming, bathing; links to other organizations and information sources (such as insurance resources and tips on writing appeal letters, Oley's travel and hospitalization packet); a clinician directory (yet to come); and much more.[15]

Learn Intestinal Failure Tele-ECHO

The Oley Foundation is on the advisory board of the newly launched (2019) Learn Intestinal Failure Tele-ECHO (LIFT-ECHO). LIFT-ECHO is a collaborative program that allows clinicians to present their patients' symptoms to a board of specialists, who then suggest to the clinician tests they could run and steps they could take during treatment. It allows clinicians to treat their patients locally, so the patient does not have to spend time and money traveling or uprooting to find a specialist. LIFT-ECHO holds virtual clinics twice monthly, where clinicians present cases related to IF (Dahl R, Oley Foundation FY 2018 and FY Q1 2019 reports, unpublished).

Awareness and Advocacy

Oley spreads their mission by exhibiting at and attending meetings nationwide, held by professional associations, home care companies, other not-for-profit organizations, and hospital programs. In 2019, Oley exhibited at the American Society for Parenteral and Enteral Nutrition (ASPEN) Science and Practice Conference in Phoenix, Arizona; the National Home Infusion Association conference in Orlando, Florida; the 6th International Pediatric Feeding Disorder Conference in Glendale, Arizona; the United Ostomy Associations of America conference in Philadelphia, Pennsylvania; the Association for Vascular Access conference in Las Vegas, Nevada; the Infusion Nurses Society conference in San Diego, California; and several ASPEN chapter meetings (Dahl R, Oley Foundation FY 2018 and FY Q1 2019 reports, unpublished).

Oley collaborates with multiple groups, such as the Digestive Disease National Coalition (DDNC), National Board of Nutrition Support Certification, Patients and Providers for Medical Nutrition Equity Coalition, and the Food and Drug Administration, to advocate on behalf of patients in need of nutritional supplements, like HPEN, and their families. With DDNC and other groups, Oley members and staff visit elected officials to represent Oley members' needs and circumstances and to put a face to HPEN therapy (Dahl R, Oley Foundation FY 2018 and FY Q1 2019 reports, unpublished).

Ambassadors

Oley Ambassadors are volunteers who have experience receiving or caring for a receiver of HPEN.[16] One Oley member said about the Oley Ambassadors:

"When I needed support the most, Oley paired me with someone who would become a lifelong friend. My ambassador not only helped me stay sane while navigating the g-tube world and all its ups and downs, she instilled hope and courage in me when our other child ended up on TPN, suddenly. The positive ripples of the support Oley provided to me still resonate today. Friendships like these are one in a million. So is Oley !(Stacie P to Lisa Metzger, Personal communication, May 28, 2019)"

Online Forum

The Oley-Inspire Forum is an online resource that connects HPEN consumers with one another through instant messaging. Available through the Oley Web site (www/oley.org/Forum), the forum allows consumers and caregivers to ask and answer questions and give and receive advice in a wide range of topics, including "Family and friends," "Home IV feeding," "Home tube feeding," and a "Spouses only" page. Clinicians are asked not to comment on posts, and consumers/caregivers are asked not to offer medical advice.[17]

Equipment and Supply Exchange Program

The cost of HEN can add up, even when insurance does cover it. In many instances, it is not covered, or the copays are significant. For this reason, Oley coordinates the exchange of new, nonprescription supplies (eg, syringes, feeding bags, extension tubing, and so on) from consumers who no longer need them to those who do, but may not be able to afford them under their insurance. The person receiving the supplies is responsible for paying for shipping, but the recipient incurs no other expenses associated with the program (Dahl R, Oley Foundation FY 2018 and FY Q1 2019 reports, unpublished).

FINDING RESOURCES

The organizations listed (including the Oley Foundation) represent a few of the many that offer programs and resources for people with IF. Professional and consumer groups are included here:

- Oley Foundation (www.oley.org)
- American Society for Parenteral and Enteral Nutrition (ASPEN) (www.nutritioncare.org)
- Association of Gastrointestinal Motility Disorders (AGMD) (www.agmdhope.org)
- AuSPEN (www.auspen.org.au)
- Caregiver Action Network (caregiveraction.org)
- Crohn's and Colitis Foundation (CCF) (www.crohnscolitisfoundation.org)
- European Society for Clinical Nutrition and Metabolism (www.ESPEN.org)

- Gastroparesis Patient Association for Cures and Treatment (G-PACT) (www.g-pact.org)
- Global Genes (www.globalgenes.org)
- International Alliance of Patient Organisations for Chronic Intestinal Failure and Home Artificial Nutrition (PACIFHAN) (pacifhan.org)
- International Foundation for Gastrointestinal Disorders (IFFGD) (www.iffgd.org)
- MitoAction (www.mitoaction.org)
- National Organization for Rare Disorders (NORD) (www.rarediseases.org)
- Parent to Parent USA (www.p2pusa.org)
- Parenteral Nutrition Down Under (PNDU) (pndu.org)
- PINNT (organization for HPEN consumers in the UK) (www.pinnt.org)
- United Ostomy Associations of America (www.ostomy.org)

(See www.oley.org/general/recommended_links.asp for the most up-to-date listing of Web sites that may be of interest to the HPEN community.)

SUMMARY

Understanding the psychosocial needs of HPEN consumers can be difficult for clinicians, which is why I (Julie) jumped at the opportunity to write this. As someone formerly on HPN and still on HEN, it is easier for me to explain and relay the value of being part of a support group, specifically the Oley Foundation, to others like me.

One could fill a book with all of the benefits the Oley Foundation provides to its members, as many people have testified. With the information provided, I will leave it up to the reader to decide: Is the Oley Foundation "just" a typical support group?

REFERENCES

1. Pironi L, Arends J, Bozzetti F, et al. ESPEN guidelines on chronic intestinal failure in adults. Clin Nutr 2016;35(2):247.
2. Pironi L, Arends J, Baxter J, et al. ESPEN endorsed recommendations. Definition and classification of intestinal failure in adults. Clin Nutr 2015;34(2):171–2.
3. Nelson EL, Yadrich DM, Thompson N, et al. Telemedicine support groups for home parenteral nutrition users. Nutr Clin Pract 2017;32(6):789–98.
4. Mundi MS, Pattinson A, McMahon MT, et al. Prevalence of home parenteral and enteral nutrition in the United States. Nutr Clin Pract 2017;32(6):799–805.
5. Chopy K, Winkler M, Schwartz-Barcott D, et al. A qualitative study of perceived value of membership in the Oley Foundation by home parenteral and enteral nutrition consumers. JPEN J Parenter Enteral Nutr 2015;39(4):426–33.
6. Metzger LC, Bishop J, Howard L. Support groups. In: Duggan PC, Gura KM, Jaksic T, editors. Clinical management of intestinal failure. Boca Raton (FL): CRC Press; 2012. p. 499–504.
7. Howard L, Ament M, Fleming CR, et al. Current use and clinical outcome of home parenteral and enteral nutrition therapies in the United States. Gastroenterology 1995;109(2):355–65.
8. Merriam-Webster. Support group. Available at: merriam.webster.com. Accessed May 31, 2019.
9. The Oley Foundation. Affiliation with Oley Foundation improves patient outcomes. Available at: www.oley.org/lifelineoutcomes. Accessed May 28, 2019.
10. Smith C, Curtas S, Werkowitch M, et al. Home parenteral nutrition: does affiliation with a national support and educational organization improve patient outcomes? JPEN J Parenter Enteral Nutr 2002;26(3):159–63.

11. Kelly DG, Bishop J, Johnson H. Meeting the unmet needs of home parenteral and enteral nutrition consumers: education, networking, and support. In: DiBaise JK, Parrish CR, Thompson JS, editors. Short bowel syndrome practical approach to management. Boca Raton (FL): CRC Press; 2016. p. 367–72.
12. The Oley Foundation. Remember Kay Oldenburg. LifelineLetter 2019;40(3):8.
13. The Oley Foundation. Member testimonials. Available at: www.oley.org/Testimonials. Accessed May 30, 2019.
14. The Oley Foundation. Webinars. Available at: www.oley.org/webinars. Accessed May 30, 2019.
15. Interview with Roslyn Dahl, communications and development director, The Oley Foundation, June 4, 2019.
16. The Oley Foundation. Welcome Ambassadors. Available at: www.oley.org/WelcomeAmbassadors. Accessed May 30, 2019.
17. Inspire. The Oley Foundation. Available at: www.inspire.com/groups/oley-foundation. Accessed May 30, 2019.

UNITED STATES POSTAL SERVICE® Statement of Ownership, Management, and Circulation (All Periodicals Publications Except Requester Publications)

1. Publication Title	2. Publication Number	3. Filing Date
GASTROENTEROLOGY CLINICS OF NORTH AMERICA	000 – 279	9/18/19

4. Issue Frequency	5. Number of Issues Published Annually	6. Annual Subscription Price
MAR, JUN, SEP, DEC	4	$351.00

7. Complete Mailing Address of Known Office of Publication (Not printer) (Street, city, county, state, and ZIP+4®)

ELSEVIER INC.
230 Park Avenue, Suite 800
New York, NY 10169

Contact Person
STEPHEN R. BUSHING

Telephone (Include area code)
215-239-3688

8. Complete Mailing Address of Headquarters or General Business Office of Publisher (Not printer)

ELSEVIER INC.
230 Park Avenue, Suite 800
New York, NY 10169

9. Full Names and Complete Mailing Addresses of Publisher, Editor, and Managing Editor (Do not leave blank)

Publisher (Name and complete mailing address)

TAYLOR BALL, ELSEVIER INC.
1600 JOHN F KENNEDY BLVD. SUITE 1800
PHILADELPHIA, PA 19103-2899

Editor (Name and complete mailing address)

KERRY HOLLAND, ELSEVIER INC.
1600 JOHN F KENNEDY BLVD. SUITE 1800
PHILADELPHIA, PA 19103-2899

Managing Editor (Name and complete mailing address)

PATRICK MANLEY, ELSEVIER INC.
1600 JOHN F KENNEDY BLVD. SUITE 1800
PHILADELPHIA, PA 19103-2899

10. Owner (Do not leave blank. If the publication is owned by a corporation, give the name and address of the corporation immediately followed by the names and addresses of all stockholders owning or holding 1 percent or more of the total amount of stock. If not owned by a corporation, give the names and addresses of the individual owners. If owned by a partnership or other unincorporated firm, give its name and address as well as those of each individual owner. If the publication is published by a nonprofit organization, give its name and address.)

Full Name	Complete Mailing Address
WHOLLY OWNED SUBSIDIARY OF REED/ELSEVIER, US HOLDINGS	1600 JOHN F KENNEDY BLVD. SUITE 1800 PHILADELPHIA, PA 19103-2899

11. Known Bondholders, Mortgagees, and Other Security Holders Owning or Holding 1 Percent or More of Total Amount of Bonds, Mortgages, or Other Securities. If none, check box ► ☐ None

Full Name	Complete Mailing Address
N/A	

12. Tax Status (For completion by nonprofit organizations authorized to mail at nonprofit rates) (Check one)
The purpose, function, and nonprofit status of this organization and the exempt status for federal income tax purposes:
☒ Has Not Changed During Preceding 12 Months
☐ Has Changed During Preceding 12 Months (Publisher must submit explanation of change with this statement)

PS Form 3526, July 2014 [Page 1 of 4 (see instructions page 4)]   PSN: 7530-01-000-9931   PRIVACY NOTICE: See our privacy policy on www.usps.com.

---

13. Publication Title			14. Issue Date for Circulation Data Below
GASTROENTEROLOGY CLINICS OF NORTH AMERICA			JUNE 2019

15. Extent and Nature of Circulation			Average No. Copies Each Issue During Preceding 12 Months	No. Copies of Single Issue Published Nearest to Filing Date
a. Total Number of Copies (Net press run)			217	219
b. Paid Circulation (By Mail and Outside the Mail)	(1)	Mailed Outside-County Paid Subscriptions Stated on PS Form 3541 (Include paid distribution above nominal rate, advertiser's proof copies, and exchange copies)	81	86
	(2)	Mailed In-County Paid Subscriptions Stated on PS Form 3541 (Include paid distribution above nominal rate, advertiser's proof copies, and exchange copies)	0	0
	(3)	Paid Distribution Outside the Mails Including Sales Through Dealers and Carriers, Street Vendors, Counter Sales, and Other Paid Distribution Outside USPS®	60	73
	(4)	Paid Distribution by Other Classes of Mail Through the USPS (e.g., First-Class Mail®)	0	0
c. Total Paid Distribution (Sum of 15b (1), (2), (3), and (4))		►	141	159
d. Free or Nominal Rate Distribution (By Mail and Outside the Mail)	(1)	Free or Nominal Rate Outside-County Copies included on PS Form 3541	60	42
	(2)	Free or Nominal Rate In-County Copies Included on PS Form 3541	0	0
	(3)	Free or Nominal Rate Copies Mailed at Other Classes Through the USPS (e.g., First-Class Mail)	0	0
	(4)	Free or Nominal Rate Distribution Outside the Mail (Carriers or other means)	0	0
e. Total Free or Nominal Rate Distribution (Sum of 15d (1), (2), (3) and (4))		►	60	42
f. Total Distribution (Sum of 15c and 15e)		►	201	201
g. Copies not Distributed (See Instructions to Publishers #4 (page 83))		►	16	18
h. Total (Sum of 15f and g)		►	217	219
i. Percent Paid (15c divided by 15f times 100)		►	70.15%	79.1%

* If you are claiming electronic copies, go to line 16 on page 3. If you are not claiming electronic copies, skip to line 17 on page 3.

16. Electronic Copy Circulation		Average No. Copies Each Issue During Preceding 12 Months	No. Copies of Single Issue Published Nearest to Filing Date
a. Paid Electronic Copies	►		
b. Total Paid Print Copies (Line 15c) + Paid Electronic Copies (Line 16a)	►		
c. Total Print Distribution (Line 15f) + Paid Electronic Copies (Line 16a)	►		
d. Percent Paid (Both Print & Electronic Copies) (16b divided by 16c × 100)	►		

☒ I certify that 50% of all my distributed copies (electronic and print) are paid above a nominal price.

17. Publication of Statement of Ownership
☒ If the publication is a general publication, publication of this statement is required. Will be printed in the DECEMBER 2019 issue of this publication.   ☐ Publication not required.

18. Signature and Title of Editor, Publisher, Business Manager, or Owner

STEPHEN R. BUSHING - INVENTORY DISTRIBUTION CONTROL MANAGER

Stephen R. Bushing   Date 9/18/19

I certify that all information furnished on this form is true and complete. I understand that anyone who furnishes false or misleading information on this form or who omits material or information requested on the form may be subject to criminal sanctions (including fines and imprisonment) and/or civil sanctions (including civil penalties).

PS Form 3526, July 2014 (Page 3 of 4)   PRIVACY NOTICE: See our privacy policy on www.usps.com.

Moving?

Make sure your subscription moves with you!

To notify us of your new address, find your **Clinics Account Number** (located on your mailing label above your name), and contact customer service at:

Email: journalscustomerservice-usa@elsevier.com

800-654-2452 (subscribers in the U.S. & Canada)
314-447-8871 (subscribers outside of the U.S. & Canada)

Fax number: 314-447-8029

Elsevier Health Sciences Division
Subscription Customer Service
3251 Riverport Lane
Maryland Heights, MO 63043

*To ensure uninterrupted delivery of your subscription, please notify us at least 4 weeks in advance of move.

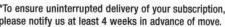

Printed and bound by CPI Group (UK) Ltd, Croydon, CR0 4YY

03/10/2024

01040477-0016